Love

"Come out of the circle of time
And into the circle of Love" -- Rumi

Love–that feeling of being one with another.
The collapsing of the separate self.
Warm rainbow liquid flowing, finding its way,
Embracing all that it touches, moving, moved by another.
Enlivened resonate energy,
Reverberating, pulsating, echoing, reflecting,
Yes, yes to all that is,
Swirling galaxies, that is me, smallest microbes, that is me,
Tell me, where are the borders of my life?
Of your life?
Where do I end and you begin?
Beyond Illusion, I ask you, are we truly one with all that is?
Are we the subject, object of our work,
Disappearing, melding – inside, outside, observer, observed – one?

Throw a blanket of love over our unknowing to warm our spirits,
So that we may move forward in wonder of all that unfolds before us.

ECODIET

TONI TONEY

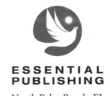

**ESSENTIAL
PUBLISHING**

North Palm Beach, FL
www.essentialpublishing.org

Essential Publishing, Inc.
378 Northlake Boulevard, Suite 109
North Palm Beach, FL 33408
www.essentialpublishing.org
(866) 770-1916

Copyright © 2013 Toni Toney

Revised Edition
ISBN 978-0-9890018-0-9
Library of Congress Control Number: 2013932888

Special Edition
ISBN 978-0-9890018-1-6
Library of Congress Control Number: 2013932887

First paperback edition published 2011
First revised paperback edition published 2013
First special edition paperback published 2013

Front cover design by Eija Strogard and Essential Publishing
Layout design by Jeri Monastero

PRINTED IN THE U.S.A.

This publication was printed by a Certified Green Printer in the United States of America, providing jobs for American workers. It was also printed, with the health of the environment in mind, on recycled paper and with vegetable-based inks, and Toni Toney is planting more trees than were required to print this publication through *Cooling the Planet.*

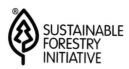

Man did not weave the web of life...he is merely a strand in it.
Whatever he does to the web, he does to himself.

—Chief Seattle

ABOUT THE AUTHOR

Toni Toney is an Internal Environmentalist who earned her "master's degree" from the highest possible school of learning: Nature! The *EcoDiet* food program is the one that Toni subscribed to when medicine failed to help her. Her purpose in writing this book is that it might help the reader, too. The author does not subscribe to the readily accepted viewpoint of "disease," but rather views pain and suffering as an internal environment out of balance with nature and the natural order of things. She encourages us to become an internal environmentalist by taking responsibility for the health and sustainability of one's own internal environment. She also encourages us to become an ecotarian—one who lives and eats for the sustainability of the body as well as the sustainability of the earth and all of its inhabitants. *EcoDiet* is the result of Toni's thirty years' experience working as an Internal Environmentalist and Natural Food Chef for clients around the globe who are suffering from what she calls an ecological breakdown, or looking for a more ecologically balanced, holistic way of living. She is the forerunner of the *Ecotarian Revolution* and is asking others to join her in the quest to "be the change we want to see in the world" and, then, inspire others to do the same!

ACKNOWLEDGMENTS

When walking the journey of life, we never walk alone. There are people who join us along the way who influence our lives more than others. There are also experiences we have along the way that influence our tomorrows more than others. Much of what I have learned about food and nutrition did not come from college textbooks or degree programs. It was born out of a "real-life" experience, acquired by my need to understand why I was sick and why medicine failed to help me. Over the years, I have traveled worldwide and studied extensively in search of answers. This book was written from the insights I gleaned regarding how the human body thrives and how it becomes sick and prematurely dies. My gratitude runs deep for all who influenced my path during my search for the truth.

I want to begin by thanking my two children, Bill and Kim, who sparked my driving force toward change. To my daughter-in-law, Halli Toney, and son-in-law, Josh Horn. To their children and my grandchildren, Camryn, Dayton, and Siera.

To Taylor Hay, for introducing me to healthy eating and taking me into my first health food store—Rainbow Blossom in Louisville, Kentucky.

To you who have taught me well.

To the many physicians I worked with throughout the years, the ones who hold to the Hippocratic principles. To Hippocrates, the father of medicine—and the greatest physician of his time—who believed in the natural healing process of rest, a good diet, sunlight, fresh air, and cleanliness and taught that there are no patients, only students.

To Dr. Ted Morter, Jr., founder of Morter Health System in Rogers, Arkansas, and creator of the Bio-Energetic Synchronization Technique (BEST), for the various health weekends I attended at your clinic, which changed my life forever and set the foundation for my life's purpose.

To Dr. Thomas Rau, Chief Medical Director of the Paracelsus Clinic in Switzerland and founder of Paracelsus Biological Medicine, for the many insights you shared with me about human health and the biological terrain during my month-long stay at your clinic.

To Dr. Richard Anderson, founder of Arise & Shine and author of *Cleanse & Purify Thyself,* for the knowledge you shared with me throughout the years about cleansing and restoring our intestinal terrain.

To Dr. Robert Morse, author of *The Detox Miracle Sourcebook,* for teaching me the anatomical truth behind our natural diet being that of a fruit eater. Understanding your detox program changed me forever.

To Dr. Michael Ryce, founder of Heartland Teaching and Retreat Center in Theodosia, Missouri, and author of *Why Is This Happening to Me, Again*, for the six months I spent at your center attending your classes on how to truly forgive.

To Lorne Label, M.D., for taking the time while vacationing in Africa to read my manuscript and write a foreword to this book.

To Dr. Howard Cohn, one of the founders of *SevenPoint2*™: *The Alkaline Company,* for believing in *EcoDiet* and writing such a magnificent introduction to this book, and for creating the transformational alkaline products of the century. These products will soon be in the hands of millions.

To the many editors who evolved this book into what it is today. Thank you to Lynn Pentz, Dr. Michael Ryce, Shirley Bennett, Carolyn Dawson, Sheridan Hill, and Linda Roberts. I especially want to thank Irma Nippert who diligently "hung in there" with me for months at my home as I gleaned insights I knew would change the way we think about food and natural feeding.

I am also in deep gratitude to Essential Publishing and Publisher Morghĕan Ó Conghalaigh for engaging in this life-changing project with me. You saw the vision, as I did, and said "yes" to make sure the information in this book gets out to the world. Working with Brian's team of editors has been a joyful intensity. Thank you Michele Poff, for your amazing editorial brilliance; you have truly been a joy to work with, and to Managing Editor Lynn Komlenic—mere words can hardly express the gratitude I want to extend to you. You have taken *EcoDiet* to new heights of awareness, which will help all who read delve deeper into understanding their natural design and natural ways of eating. I will forever be grateful for the many revisions that you made to make *EcoDiet*—the book I knew it could one day become.

To the many friends and family members who gave me lots of insightful feedback and encouragement along the way. Thank you to Dr. Richard Anderson, Gail Batke, Kavita Daswani, Neville Raymond, Irene Newman, Jack Malone, Judith Johnson, Cheri Bowers, Ken Cadigan, Steve Tilton, Dino DeFilippi, Leonard Farrell, Don Tolman, Joe Piscateli, Gwendolyn Morton, Bill Bowers, Kathryn Phelps, Karen Ormstead, Chuck Peters, Summer Kolesar, James Taylor, Mary Anne Wise, Helene Abrams, David Giller, Sondra Ray, Mark Sullivan, and Karol Avalon.

To Jodie Rhodes with Jodie Rhodes Literary Agency, who believed that this manuscript should be "out there" and supported me in every way possible.

To all my friends on the island of Patmos in Greece.

To Eija Storgard for helping to create such a magnificent book cover design.

To Heli and Tony for introducing me to Eija and Essential Publishing.

To my sponsors Dr. Richard Anderson and Arise & Shine, Carolyn Dawson, Gwendolyn and Philip Morton, Roxanne Bartels, and Paul Morton.

To Art Schwab, for being my most trusted friend throughout the years, and for believing in me and supporting me in every way.

To James Menzel Joseph for his loving offering of his painting and poem at the front of this book, which sets the tone for *EcoDiet* so eloquently and perfectly.

CONTENTS

PART ONE
OUR INTERNAL ENVIRONMENT
How We Thrive and How We Die

PART TWO
ECODIET
The New Dietary Revolution

PART THREE
THE ECODIET PROGRAM
How to Fuel Your Body for High Performance

FOREWORD
by Lorne Label, MD, MBA, FAAN

Toni Toney's new book, *EcoDiet,* provides a unique and refreshing approach to our health and how it interfaces with the health of our planet. Toni Toney uniquely reveals various interlinking depictions of the human body and the earth and how we are polluting and destroying them both in much the same way. Simultaneously, we are provided an intuitively simple, yet sophisticated approach to both the workings and failings of the ecological world around and within us. Although the thrust of the book is proper nourishment for our bodies, we also learn that ecological balance creates health. Imbalance creates disease; not just for us, but for our planet at large.

Using both hard and soft science, Toni Toney thoroughly elaborates on the ecological equilibrium of the human body and the earth we inhabit. She explores the health and diseases of our bodies in a new way, comparing and contrasting them to the health and diseases of our planet. She presents an innovative insight into the types of food we feed into our internal environment and how an acid diet loaded with toxic chemicals creates a type of internal acid rain. She then offers a unique and easy-to-follow explanation of the value and procedure involved in measuring the pH of the body's internal waters to see if acid rain is negatively effecting the environment of the body.

We have long known that the earth has been devastated by acid rain and various other environmental pollutants, but what we haven't known is that the human body has been devastated by this internal acid rain caused by ingesting acid food, acid air, and acid water. The acidic wastes from chemical additives and processed foods may be the common denominator in many degenerative diseases. We know that in many medical conditions, the accumulated acidic waste causes organ damage.

Though still somewhat controversial in the field of medical studies, the information regarding the acid/alkaline balance and its involvement with disease is both intriguing and plausible. The theory behind the alkaline diet is that the human body is alkaline by design; and thus our diet should support maintaining a blood pH between 7.35-7.45. Since all foods that we eat, digest, and metabolize produce either an acid or alkaline base (bicarbonate) in the blood, our diet should be alkaline-producing.

In the past, it was questioned whether acid-producing foods actually promote the loss of essential minerals such as potassium, magnesium, calcium, and sodium as the body tries to restore equilibrium. In the October 2001 *European Journal of Nutrition,* Dr. Katherine Tucker wrote *"The Acid-Base Hypothesis: Diet and Bone in the Framingham Osteoporosis Study,"* supporting the role of base-forming foods and nutrients in bone maintenance. More evidence-based studies in this area will be worthwhile. What medical science does know, however, is that certain foods have substantial anti-cancer effects, while others are important in preventing the formation of calcium kidney stones, osteoporosis, and age-related muscle wasting.

EcoDiet is much more than just another book on how to eat in an acid/alkaline type fashion. Toni has been teaching her internal environment dietary principles to students across the world for decades. Finally, she has assimilated her body of knowledge and described it in a straightforward approach. She explains why certain foods create a type of environmental SOS signal, a pre-disaster internal global warning that we must learn to heed. There are extensive lists and charts providing exact information of both the best and worst types of food we should or shouldn't be burning for fuel into our internal environment. Proper preparation of these food groups into delicious dishes is another highlight of this book.

In an almost cookbook-type fashion, the first part of *EcoDiet* lays the groundwork for the most ideal diet, both theoretically and practically, that we should all strive for. The last part is the *EcoDiet* program that features lots of wonderful recipes.

Though the U.S. government's 2005 *Dietary Guidelines for Americans (My Pyramid)* does break down the five food groups into grains, vegetables, fruit, milk, meat and beans, the specifics are vague. There is neither information on the actual contents of each food group nor description of the best and worst of the foods. For example, under the food group *vegetables*, the recommendations include "eat more dark green and orange vegetables and dried beans or peas include fresh, frozen or canned chopped vegetables." The suggestions under the food group *fruit*, state "choose a variety of fresh, frozen, canned or dried fruit."

Clearly, the government's recommendations are vague, not helpful, and to some extent potentially unhealthy. Anyone trying to understand the best foods to eat and how to prepare them is left stranded. Common sense should tell us that recommending canned fruit with all its sweeteners is not the healthiest approach.

As pointed out in *EcoDiet,* there are large varieties of healthy fruits and vegetables to choose from with, surprisingly, other types (potentially our favorite foods) that would be best to avoid. The 2005 *MyPyramid* leaves that information unclear. So do many other diet books on the market. Toni Toney clarifies the information for us.

This book is not a panacea. It is a call to action. It will make you think about how the internal environment of the body is a reflection of the outer, which will most likely change your approach to the kind of foods you eat. In fact, I believe it presents one of the easiest guidelines to follow in keeping the pH balance correct for excellent health.

Toni Toney's message throughout this book is: We are one. The earth reflects us and we reflect the earth. What is internal to our planet is our internal village. What is external to our planet reflects our external village. Toni says that to shift our planet's environmental crisis around, we need to "be the change" and shift the crisis within ourselves.

I invite you to join us in this amazing crusade for health: a healthy body and a healthy planet. The time is now for each of us to "Answer the Call."

So join Toni Toney's *EcoDiet*—The New Dietary Revolution!

Dr. Lorne Label

Lorne Label, MD, MBA, FAAN
Associate Clinical Professor of Neurology
David Geffin School of Medicine, UCLA, Los Angeles, CA

INTRODUCTION
by Howard Cohn, DC

It's been said that there are no accidents in the world. It is not an accident that you are holding this transformational book, *EcoDiet,* by Toni Toney in your hands right now. In this book, Toni Toney takes us on a journey of personal discovery and deep internal searching for truth. It's written from personal experience from someone who was searching for answers as to why she had become extremely ill—seemingly out of nowhere—and had almost died. Her search took her all over the world as well as to the origins and history of how and why our internal and external environments have become what they've become.

With well over twenty years of experience as a nutritional researcher, environmentalist, and organic whole food gourmet chef and restaurateur, Toni shares with us what she has learned, which is that an alkaline environment is absolutely everything—for the outer environment as well as our internal environments. The food we are burning for fuel sets the stage for health and longevity or disease and premature death. It's time to wake up! How we are treating our earth is how we are treating ourselves.

In the *EcoDiet,* Toni eloquently demystifies and ties the mirror that exists between human physiology and the realities of our ecological world together. In his definitive text on human physiology entitled, *Textbook of Medical Physiology,* Arthur Guyton, MD states, "The first step to maintaining health is to alkalize the body. The cells of a healthy body are alkaline while the cells of a diseased body are acidic. Since our bodies do not manufacture alkalinity, we must supply the alkalinity from an outside source to keep us from being acidic and dying." Like most doctors who were assigned Guyton's textbook for human physiology classes, I read it, studied it, and was tested on it, but never really applied it. It was only when I started seeing patients, and observing the remarkable difference in the health and healing of those who led an alkaline lifestyle and those who didn't, that the truth of that knowledge really landed.

So, why is this book so important? If we want to save our planet for our children and grandchildren, we must first save ourselves. A drowning person cannot save a drowning person. Even when we board an airplane, we are told to secure our own life mask first *before* assisting others. For things to change, we must change. In this book, we not only learn why to do it, we learn how to do it. Toni educates us and holds our hand every step of the way.

There's a famous Chinese Proverb which states "Don't wait until you're thirsty, to dig a well," which means that it's a whole lot easier to stay well than it is to get well. A good portion of our world will have a fatal heart attack as their first symptom of heart disease. Science has shown us that a tumor can be growing for up to eight years in a woman's breast before it is even visible on a mammogram.

This book may very well be your wake up call. Do not reach for the snooze button, the time is now! The Alkaline Movement is here. It is not a fad; it is the truth.

> "Truth is, by nature, self-evident; as soon as you remove
> the cobwebs of ignorance that surround it, it shines clear."
> —Mahatma Gandhi

It takes just one light to illuminate even the darkest of rooms. I believe that this timely message, given to us by Toni Toney in the *EcoDiet* is the light that will lead us and our planet back to health.

Today, tonight, someone, somewhere, will take a knee in prayer, hoping that someone, somewhere will share with them an answer to the suffering of a family member, friend, loved one, or themselves. This book and its life-altering message, when implemented as it is designed, may very well be the answer to the prayers of many. Live its message, share it and change the world.

> "You must be the change you wish to see in the world."
> —Mahatma Gandhi

Yours in health,

Howard Cohn, DC
Founder and Director, Cohn Health Institute
Chief Product Officer, *SevenPoint2*™: *The Alkaline Company*

PART ONE

OUR INTERNAL ENVIRONMENT
How We Thrive and How We Die!

Chapter 1

HOW I ALMOST DIED

We are not separate from our Creator, nature,
anyone, or anything outside of us.

This book has taken me a very long time to write. Page one was written thirty-three years ago, when I got sick and almost died. My body had been sending me S-O-S signals for years, but I didn't "Answer the Call!" I was too busy with my real estate career and raising a family to listen, or so I thought. I just kept turning a deaf ear to my symptoms with aspirins and pharmaceutical drugs, ignoring the warning signals. Like planet Earth, I was in the midst of an environmental crisis. A type of global warming was threatening my very life.

I woke up one morning drenched in a feverish sweat. After collapsing to the floor, I was rushed to the hospital. Following a series of blood tests, I was admitted to an isolation room due to a dangerously low white-blood-cell count. For days, my white-blood-cell count continued to drop, despite many rounds of the strongest intravenous antibiotics possible. Even the most acclaimed immunologists studying my case had no clue to the cause and, therefore, no cure for my problem. They simply blamed my declining white-blood-cell count on some mysterious germ and told me that if my white-blood-cell count didn't start to increase soon, I may not live.

Intense fear had me in its grip. I didn't want to die. I had two young children who needed their mother. Yet, I had overheard the doctors explain to my family outside my door that they needed to prepare for the worst. I heard frightened pleas and hopelessness in my family's voices as they questioned medicine's best answers.

The silence of the long night held me captive. I was afraid to sleep, stricken with the terror that I might never wake up. I wanted to live—if not for me, for my children. But the high fever was relentless and, in my exhaustion, I could sense my hold on life fading away.

Isolated from everyone in my sterile hospital room, I closed my eyes, finally willing to slip beyond the world of my physical existence. That's when I heard a still, small voice speak inside of me:

There is only one problem, ever: The illusion of separation.
Focus on your breath and you will live!

For hours, I kept my attention on my breath. I sensed a presence within me that was incomprehensible to my human mind. A wave of determination to live rushed all through me. Something deep inside of me had shifted; I felt it. I could sense my oneness with my Creator, nature, everything, and everyone around me. I was not separate from anything or anyone, as I had once believed.

Completely surrendered to this newfound presence within me, I fell asleep, and woke to an entirely new day. After another round of blood tests, my doctor came in with astonishing news: "During my twenty-some-odd years of practicing medicine, I've never seen a recovery quite like this. Your white-blood-cell count is almost normal. I just wish I had an explanation for it all."

I replied, "I'm glad you don't—you might just explain away my miracle!" While I was relieved to know that I was going to live, every joint in my body hurt.

HIPPOCRATES: THE FATHER OF MEDICINE

As fate would have it, Taylor, my friend and real estate broker, stopped by to see me and told me that a few years earlier he too had had a brush with death. Shortly thereafter, he shifted his eating habits from the extremely acidic Standard American Diet (SAD), which is high in processed foods, meat, dairy products, refined grains, sugary desserts and drinks, to a whole-foods, plant-based alkaline diet high in fruits and vegetables, and experienced what others would call a miracle. Knowing that I had been eating the highly acidic Standard American Diet, he encouraged me to do the same.

Taylor looked up at my IV drip and told me that Hippocrates, the ancient Greek physician, believed that the main duty of a physician was to empower a sick person to heal themself through guidance, education and support. He did not believe that physicians, per se, healed patients; he believed that the body has an innate intelligence to heal itself and will do so, *when provided the proper conditions.* Hence, he did not consider or relate to the ill as *patients*, but rather as *students* whose role was to learn how health is achieved, and to adopt health-giving practices. Physicians, therefore, assisted students in their understanding of health as a natural effect of *balance*, and disease as a result of *imbalance*; they imparted knowledge of the body's systems and functions, and prescribed tools (herbs, foods, exercise, therapeutic treatments like baths and massage, and the like), and then stood by to allow nature to do its job.

Taylor said, "I believe Hippocrates would turn over in his grave if he could see how the physicians of our time are using drugs as medicine and treating people as patients instead of using food as medicine and treating you as a student. So, if you *truly* want to turn your health crisis around, you need to check yourself out of 'man's' hospital and check yourself into 'nature's' hospital."

He paused for a moment then said, "Our Creator never intended for us to be separate from nature or the foods that were designed to keep us connected to our Divine nature." He went on to quote Hippocrates' famous statement: *Let food be your medicine and medicine be your food.*

THE INTERNAL TERRAIN THEORY

As Taylor was leaving, he handed me some articles on the internal terrain theory. I read how Antoine Béchamp, a nineteenth-century contemporary of Louis Pasteur, recognized that when the internal environment of the human body is in a state of balance, germs do not have a breeding ground. Pasteur and Béchamp each conducted research into the cause of disease. They even worked side by side, though they came to very different conclusions.

Pasteur believed that the interior of the human body was sterile and static like a spotlessly clean Petri dish. He believed that the cell was the elementary unit of life and hypothesized that harmful airborne microbes invaded the body, attacking us from the outside, causing such physical reactions as fermentation, putrefaction, and disease. He taught that we are the prey, and the germs are the predators.

This perspective is well known today as the *germ* theory.

Béchamp, on the other hand, believed that "disease is born of us and in us." He hypothesized that the cell couldn't be the elementary unit of life because the cells of our blood and tissues contained countless microscopic living entities, which he named microzymas. These microzymas, he found, were pleomorphic—they had the ability to assume or morph into many different forms depending on the body's internal state. In a healthy body, the microzymas assisted and existed peacefully as beneficial bacteria in the natural and necessary function of fermentation (the process whereby large organic molecules are broken down to simpler molecules by microorganisms). In a diseased body, however, the microzymas morph into harmful bacteria, fungi and yeasts, and proliferate—as some doctors believe—in an attempt to remove the body of toxins, but creating additional problems in the meanwhile.

In his last book, *The Third Element of the Blood*, Béchamp said this about microzymas:

> ". . . the microzyma, whatever its origin, is a ferment; it is organized, it is living, capable of multiplying, of becoming diseased and of communicating [causing] disease. All microzyma are ferments of the same order—that is to say, they are organisms, able to produce alcohol, acetic acid, lactic acid and butyric acid... In a state of health the microzymas of the organism act harmoniously, and our life is, in every meaning of the word, a regular fermentation. In a state of disease, the microzymas do not act harmoniously, and the fermentation is disturbed; the microzymas have either changed their function or are placed in an abnormal situation by some modification of the medium."

Béchamp found that microzymas could not only change their form, but their function as well, from helpful to hostile and back again, depending on internal conditions. To his amazement, he found that microzymas were so strong that he was unable to destroy them at the highest of temperatures or with highly toxic chemicals. He even found live microzymas in limestone dating to a geologic period some sixty million years ago when the first mammals appeared on Earth.

In other words, microzymas are not only a critical part of living organisms, but they seem to be indestructible.

Indeed, Béchamp discovered that microzymas are present in the tissues and blood of all living organisms, where they remain helpful until the well-being of the body is threatened by toxic material.

It is only after our body's internal environment has long remained in a toxic state that microzymas lose their symbiotic, life-enhancing qualities and devolve into harmful bacteria, yeasts and fungus. These "bad" microzyma themselves give off toxic byproducts, further contributing to a weakened terrain, making the body more susceptible, then, to external bacteria. Uninterrupted, the internal state becomes progressively worse, accelerating the shift toward disease and death. The irony is that it is the state of our internal terrain that causes *them* to behave poorly; they are simply responding to the environment that we are creating. However—and this is the good news—Béchamp discovered that once a pristine and harmonious internal environment has been restored, that microzymas revert back into their harmless, dormant form! So, the key is to restore the balance of our internal terrain, which is my purpose in writing this book.

Béchamp concluded that the real cause of disease and death was not the so-called *germ* (as asserted by Pasteur), but rather a toxic internal environment that causes the body's typically healthy microorganisms to, in effect, behave badly. This was supported by leading nutritional experts Dr. Bernard Jensen and Mark Anderson in their book *Empty Harvest*,

> "The germ theory is still believed to be the central cause of disease because around it exists a colossal supportive infrastructure of commercial interests that built multi-billion-dollar industries based upon this theory. To the scientific satisfaction of many in the health field, it has long been disproven as the primary cause of disease. Germs are, rather, an effect of disease."

Further, Béchamp is reputed to have said, "living beings, filled with microzymas, carry within themselves the elements essential for health or for disease, for life, or for death."

His perspective, called the *internal terrain theory*, is a theory that remains highly viable today. To our detriment, however, it is still largely unaccepted by conventional medical scientists and practitioners in favor of germ theory.

Since the time that Béchamp discovered microzymas in the mid-1800s and postulated the internal terrain theory, however, a small group of dedicated scientists and advocates have studied Béchamp's work and are evolving this science to such a level that it has the potential to shake conventional medicine.

Dr. Enderlein of Germany and microbiologist Gaston Naessens of France were able to show that in addition to forming bacteria, viruses and yeasts, microzymas were also able to form parasites. Through a powerful microscope that Naessens invented himself, he was able to observe and map a cycle of sixteen different pleomorphic transmutations of *somatids*, as he termed the microzyma.

Naessens found that when our internal environment is clean and healthy, the microzymas have a healthy three-state reproduction cycle. But, when the internal environment becomes toxic, weakened or destabilized, there are thirteen other possible stages of transmutation, including conversion into unhealthy microbes. The somatids, specifically, were found to mutate through various forms that can produce bacteria, fungus, yeast, parasites, *and* viruses. Health, therefore, which can be defined as our ability to maintain a state of biochemical equilibrium free from disease, has *everything* to do with the condition of our *internal* environment.

As Béchamp established, disease occurs only when our internal environment is favorable for the growth of harmful pathogens. This is very unlike the prevailing belief in conventional medical circles today—as postulated and supported by advocates of germ theory—that diseased is caused by external pathogens, which is incorrect according to Béchamp. The correct way of thinking about disease, he posited, is that it occurs when our immune system becomes weakened, first by actions that create an unfavorable internal environment (consuming non-nutritive foods, smoking, drug use, etc.), and then further weakened by internal organisms like microzyma, which are typically helpful to the body but become pathogenic (capable of producing disease) when exposed to a toxic internal environment. We then *become* much more susceptible to and incapable of dealing successfully with external pathogens when we are exposed to them.

Thus, the internal terrain theory reflects a very important message: our health begins and ends with us. By nourishing our bodies with proper nutrients through life-sustaining foods, clean water and air, sunshine, beneficial thoughts and relationships, exercise and employment in service to others—all of the essential building blocks for a healthy human life—we have the ability to shape the health of our internal terrain, enabling our internal mechanisms to operate optimally, and live free from disease.

THE GERM: THE CAUSE, THE CURE

Even though my family thought I had become insanely delirious from the high fever, Béchamp's internal terrain theory rang true to me, so I took my friend's advice and checked myself out of the hospital.

I was full of hope!

A few hours after my arrival at home, Taylor came by with bags of organic fruits and vegetables. When he put a large juice machine on my kitchen countertop and handed me books on the healing power of food and juice fasting, I just shook my head. It all seemed so strange to me. Yet, I couldn't put the books down; I read all through the night. While reading, I could sense momentary flickers of this newfound presence within me. It was as though its guiding force kept nudging me awake, its voice saying "yes" to everything I was reading.

Because our bodies are slightly alkaline by design and fruits and vegetables are the way to keep the body's alkalinity, I decided to put my new juicer to work and juiced my way to wellness!

Needless to say, my two children rebelled when I offered them carrot juice and a bowl of fruit instead of chocolate milk and a sticky bun for breakfast the next morning. But, I was on a mission—not just to heal myself, but to make sure my children stayed healthy as well.

Work had taken a back seat. I stayed at home creating recipes my entire family could enjoy. I also read every book I could find on whole foods and natural healing.

I especially enjoyed reading about Hippocrates and his prescriptions for health. I read how he taught his students to trust in nature to heal the body, and the body to heal the mind—that they were interconnected. His prescribed medicines were whole foods, rest, fresh air, and sunlight. He also used purges, enemas, herbs, and fasting diets to evacuate toxicity from the body; the application of friction to increase circulation through massage; and the use of hot and cold water to further stimulate circulation.

I decided to follow Hippocrates' prescriptions. The more I purified myself, the more connected I felt to my Creator, nature, and everyone around me.

Then, after about ninety days, the pain had vanished. I had juiced, cleansed, eaten, and prayed my way to wellness—my internal environmental crisis had been turned around.

Some called it a miracle. I called it "a return to my natural state of being." I began to remove the cause of my illness and found the cure!

The cause: A toxic internal environment caused in part by eating the Standard America Diet high in acidifying foods such as meat, dairy, and sugar—a diet that prevents us from experiencing true health and, therefore, our true nature.

The cure: A toxic-free internal environment caused in part by eating a diet high in alkalizing whole foods, such as fruits and vegetables—a diet that makes it possible for us to connect with our true nature as compassionate, cooperative, loving beings.

With time, the more alkaline my body became, the healthier my mind became. Insights began to unfold within me that changed my life forever and prepared me for my destiny.

I began to view the world through eyes of oneness. The illusion of separation was lifting. I could see that our planet's environmental crisis and our body's environmental crisis were reflections of each other. We are destroying ourselves in the same way we are destroying our planet. We are not separate!

Albert Einstein said it best:

A human being is a part of the whole, called by us "Universe," a part limited in time and space. He experiences himself, his thoughts and feelings as something separated from the rest—a kind of optical delusion of his consciousness. This delusion is a kind of prison for us, restricting us to our personal desires and to affection for a few persons nearest to us. Our task must be to free ourselves from this prison by widening our circle of compassion to embrace all living creatures and the whole of nature in its beauty.

Take a moment and ask yourself these few questions—the same ones I had to ask myself:

- Am I really separate from my Creator, from nature, and from everything and everyone around me?

- What is this life force inside of me that knows how to repair my physical body when I work with it and not against it?

- Is it possible that my body is one with the earth?

- Is it possible that global warming and climate change are happening within me, and everyone around me—that we're all going through a type of planetary shift?

- Could the disease I've been tagged with, and the pain I feel, be the S-O-S signal my body's intelligence is sending, warning me that I am burning the wrong type of fuel in my body?

- Am I ready to "Answer the Call?"

I now know that in order for us to affect real change in the world, we are being called to be the change: to end the illusion of separation; to know that we are one with our Creator, to know that everything and everyone we see outside of us are merely a reflection of what is taking place within us.

It is time for each of us to thrive, time to put an end to our own individual environmental crisis. When we do, we will shift our planet, along with everything and everyone that "appears" to be outside of us!

Chapter 2

OUR BODY IS A LIVING ECOSYSTEM

*The condition of our internal environment
spawns life and health or death and disease.*

My desire to understand our oneness with planet Earth and how we both thrive and die took me all over the world. Over the years, I traveled extensively, visiting and studying at various holistic healing centers including the world-renowned Paracelsus Clinic in Switzerland. It was there that I began to understand more about Béchamp's internal terrain theory and how a pristine, alkaline environment is absolutely everything!

Eventually, I found my way to the Greek island of Kos and stood at the tree of Hippocrates, acknowledging the Father of Medicine for giving me nature's prescription on how to return my internal environment back into balance with its natural way of being. It was there that I began to make some very intriguing connections.

The earliest Greek philosophers saw the world around them and sought rational explanations to the origin and nature of the physical world, a philosophy that formed the foundation of Western science and natural philosophy. Central to this worldview, the Greek philosophers often divided the world into four elements: earth, air, fire, and water.

Then, through this model of the elemental world, Greek medicine took its stance: the cause and cure of illness were rooted in the larger conceptual viewpoint of the elemental world.

In essence, it became clear to me that the human body, like the planet, is a living ecosystem made up of earth, air, fire, and water—the same classical elements of the world according to ancient Greek philosophy. How we thrive and die is, in part, the same, and involves a balance of these same four elements.

EAT RIGHT FOR YOUR ELEMENTAL TYPE

Our body is truly magnificent. Like the landscapes of the earth, every tissue, every gland, every organ is an ecosystem composed of earth, air, fire, and water. If we look at things from the modern scientific perspective, we see that the same truth prevails—we are made up of the same elements as our planet. The human body is also composed of oxygen, carbon, hydrogen, and nitrogen, along with a very small amount of electrolyte minerals and trace mineral compounds.

This chart shows the percentage of each major element in our body, and the specific purpose each element serves.

Our Elemental Composition

Element	% of Body Weight	Primary Systems Requiring This Element
Oxygen	65 %	All Fluids, Bones, Teeth, Skin, Red Blood Cells, Circulation
Carbon	18 %	Teeth, Skin, Connective Tissue, Hair, Nails
Hydrogen	10 %	Blood and Cells
Nitrogen	3 %	Muscles, Cartilage, Tissues, Ligaments, Tendons, Flesh
Calcium	2 %	Bones and Teeth
Phosphorus	1 %	Blood and Brain

Derived from H. A. Harper, V. W. Rodwell, P.A. Mayes, *Review of Physiological Chemistry*, 16th ed. (Los Altos, CA: Lange Medical Publications, 1977).

There are numerous other minerals that comprise the human body, but they are in concentrations of less than 1%, so they will not be listed here. Suffice it to say, however, that *all* of these elements play a critical role in our health, and when our bodies don't get the necessary nutrients, and our elemental balance gets out of whack, disease results. So, let's visit the key elements and see what they tell us about health.

The internal environment of the human body is made up of mostly oxygen. Oxygen and hydrogen can combine to produce water. The human body is approximately 75% water, just like the earth. If the elemental foundation of our body is primarily oxygen, and oxygen is held within the structure of fluids in the body, then keeping our internal water-based components (blood, lymph, etc.) clean and our oxygen levels high must be two of the most important factors for maintaining our health.

How do we do this, you ask? Well, the key lies in pH!

pH: THE KEY TO ECOLOGICAL EQUILIBRIUM

The term pH can be a little intimidating to some when, in essence, it is actually simple. In practical terms, pH is a measure of the acidity or alkalinity of a water-based fluid. The pH scale runs from 0 to 14. A pH measurement of 7 is defined as neutral, being neither acid nor alkaline. Water with a pH measurement of less than 7 is acid—the lower the number, the more acidic the water. Any number greater than 7 is alkaline—the higher the number, the greater the alkalinity.

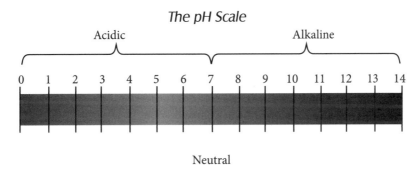

By nature, an alkaline fluid holds much more oxygen than an acidic fluid. As a solution becomes more acidic, it contains less and less oxygen and is, therefore, less able to support *life*.

As it pertains to the human body, if our internal waters are alkaline and oxygen-rich, our cells thrive; if they are acidic and oxygen-starved, and loaded with toxic waste, our cells die. Simply put, when enough of our cells die, our bodies break down, and we become ill.

Maintaining the proper pH is, then, essential for *both* health and life, and it is what this book is going to show you how to do.

Our human bodies are mildly alkaline by design (between 7.2 and 7.35) and so are the mineral residues of fruits and vegetables. This is the primary reason a plant-based alkaline diet, along with supplementing your diet with alkaline products from companies such as *SevenPoint2™: The Alkaline Company* is the foundation for building or maintaining perfect health.

So, the secret to keeping your internal environment healthy and replete with oxygen is an alkaline diet. It is that simple!

NATURAL FEEDING WITHIN ECOSYSTEMS

An ecosystem is a biological community of interdependent organisms that live symbiotically within an environment, each depending upon the other to thrive. The equilibrium of an ecosystem is delicate and any disruption, such as an unsuitable food supply or a toxic overload, can damage or destroy it.

Our earth's ecosystem consists of many interconnected ecosystems and various forms of life, such as lakes, forests, and the microscopic life of soils. Our body's ecosystems also consist of various forms of life, such as the circulatory system, organs, and the microenvironments of the cells.

The main source of energy for every ecosystem is the sun. Green plants, algae, and various other organisms capture the energy from sunlight and convert it into chemical energy that is used as fuel for the growth of living matter. The process of using the sun's energy to fuel growth is called *photosynthesis*.

Photosynthesis produces bio-fuel that is made available to living organisms through a relationship of feeding known as the food chain. In the hierarchy of the *food chain*, each group feeds on the group below it, all benefitting from the chemical energy of photosynthesis. As an example, humans benefit from the sun's energy by eating fruits from trees that are produced through photosynthesis. Animals are the same, in that they either consume plants as a primary source of fuel, or other animals that consume plants. Basically, no matter where a species lies on the food chain, if they are feeding from nature, they are consuming food that has the sun's energy.

In fact, this way of *natural feeding* can be used to divide every living creature in an ecosystem into one of three categories: *producer organisms, consumer organisms,* and *reducer organisms*. Producer organisms produce food for other species, consumer organisms consume food, and reducer organisms convert previously living creatures back into organic matter. In order for us to understand how to thrive, we must understand where we belong within the intricate, living ecosystems of the earth.

Producer Organisms

Green plants

Through the process of photosynthesis, green plants produce the food upon which *all* other life depends, which is why they are called *producer organisms*. Green plants convert the sun's energy directly into complex carbohydrates that either form the body of the green plant itself or are stored as phytonutrients in fruits, nuts, and seeds. Green plants are the foundation of the food chain. During the process of photosynthesis, carbon dioxide and water are broken down, releasing oxygen as a waste product. Photosynthesis is what maintains normal atmospheric oxygen levels for consumer organisms and all aerobic (oxygen-requiring) processes that take place within us.

Consumer Organisms

Primary Consumer Organisms

Frugivores

I am going to spend some time talking about frugivores for reasons that you are about to read. Frugivores are creatures that feed on fruit, to one degree or another. There is one group of frugivores in which I am primarily interested—a genus whose food source is primarily fruit; this group is primates. Primates are designed to feed primarily on fruit, with some seeds and green leaves; not only do they feed on this diet, they thrive on it. Now, it might not be surprising to you to hear that primates, such as apes and chimpanzees, are the type of frugivore that I just described, but it just might shake you to the bone to hear this—humans are this type of frugivore too, and a diet consisting primarily of fruits is the diet we were designed to eat!

While you may not believe what you are reading, and it will almost surely take some time for you to literally digest and assimilate this news, consider what anthropologist Katharine Milton, professor at the University of California, Berkeley asserted, which is that many characteristics of modern primates, including humans, derive from an early ancestor's practice of taking most of its food from the tropical canopy. She also notes that:

"Food eaten by humans today, especially those consumed in industrially advanced nations, bears little resemblance to the plant-based diets anthropoids (monkeys, apes and humans) have favored since their emergence."

While we are technically only 1.6% different than chimpanzees and, surprisingly, closer to them in genetic structure than a dog is to a fox, a white-handed gibbon is to a white-cheeked crested gibbon, and an Indian elephant is to an African elephant, our diets are, indeed, extremely different, especially in the case of those consuming the Standard American Diet. You will see examples of scientific evidence in forthcoming chapters supporting the fact that humans, like apes and monkeys, are predominantly fruit and plant eaters by ecological design. I also believe that you will see a growing body of evidence by researchers and scientists in the next several years to this reality and, more importantly, to its connection to the diseases that have plagued humanity for some time, and are assaulting us with greater vengeance now. Milton even goes as far to say:

"Such findings lend support to the suspicion that many health problems common in technologically advanced nations may result, at least in part, from a mismatch between the diets we now eat and those to which our bodies became adapted over millions of years."

A chimpanzee's diet is primarily fruit, comprising approximately 68%. The rest of their diet is the following: leaves 11%, seeds 7%, flowers 2%, bark 1%, pith 2%, insects 6%, and mammals 2%. As you can see, an extremely small percentage of their diet is actually uncooked, unprocessed animal flesh, insects precluded. It may also surprise you to learn that of all the ape species, only chimpanzees, bonobos (pygmy chimpanzees), and the orangutan on rare occasion have been observed eating animals flesh, the rest do not consume animals except in the form of insects as they are eating plant matter. While we are obviously not identical to chimpanzees, we are close enough to pay mind to our great physiological similarities, and how they relate particularly to food gathering, consumption and digestion, and learn from them.

Like Dr. Milton, a growing number of researchers and scientists advocate natural feeding as a solution to our chronic health problems. They argue that it is the very departure from our natural way of feeding that is causing our problems, and more of us to ask "What is the optimal diet for humans?" This is the question that I aim to answer in this book. But wait! There is another twist…

The New Frugivore—Meet the Ecotarian

While it is true that I am advocating that humans consume a diet much like our closest relative the chimpanzee, there is one difference: I do *not* advocate the consumption of meat. There are numerous reasons for this, to which I speak throughout this text. However, the primary reason is that it is not healthy or sustainable for humans or our environment. As meat consumption relates to humans, I will tell you that not only do we not have the capability of digesting meat thoroughly and properly, especially cooked animal flesh, but that meat is toxic and acidifying to our bodies, which, as you will learn later, creates a low-oxygen state, enabling pathogens (disease-causing organisms) to thrive. Equally important, is that the raising of animals for human consumption, fowl and cattle in particular, is incredibly acidifying and damaging to our earth, not to mention to our hearts.

Industrial animal farming is cruel at best: it creates numerous problems for our ecosystem and our psyche (whether we are aware of it or not), and is directly connected to the health and environmental crises that we face today. If we are to overcome the challenges that face our species and planet at large, we must have the courage to examine our current practices and be willing to discard those that are harmful to us—and other life forms—for more sensible, utilitarian solutions, which is what I am proposing in asking you to become an ecotarian. This is the new type of frugivore, one that chooses to eat by natural design, but also to not consume animal flesh, because of the suffering and disease that it causes to all life forms, including our planet.

I define an ecotarian as a person who eats for the sustainability of their body and our planet, a person who consumes consciously, recognizing our oneness with all life forms. While this might sound like spiritual nonsense to some, I truly believe that until we realize our deep interconnectedness between ourselves and other life forms, including our living planet, we cannot and will not become a healthy species, and we will miss the grandest opportunity available to us at this time in our development, which is to realize our true nature as cooperative and loving beings, and experience our full capacity as human beings. We have operated for eons as a populous desirous of domination—over one another, other life forms, and, remarkably, nature. We are losing this battle, and it is our imperative to see this if we desire true health.

If you are reading this book, I congratulate you, and ask that you reflect on this question: Do you believe that you have the best chance of achieving a healthy body if you are eating the way you were designed to eat? The answer to this question will determine how closely you examine and consider the content in this book. Trust me when I tell you this: if your answer is "Yes," then you will be one of the few who is in store for the most wonderful journey that you can imagine! Try the programs that I have outlined here and experience the results for yourself; it may just be the best thing that you ever do.

Herbivores

Animals such as deer, rabbits, and cattle are also called consumer organisms because they acquire their energy primarily from consuming grasses and leaves (foliage), and only a few fruits, nuts, and seeds.

The Difference Between Herbivores and Frugivores

It is understandable to think of humans as herbivores because we do eat vegetation—grasses and leaves. However, we are not. To confuse the matter even further, scientists say these categories (along with omnivore and carnivore) are not so easy to define, and can overlap and be subdivided. Frugivores can be viewed as a subdivision of traditional herbivore, with a more specific herbivore the other category. There are important differences between these two subcategories of herbivore. Frugivores, such as humans, consume parts of plants containing little or no cellulose, and the predominant food items for this group are plants' reproductive parts (fruit, seeds, and nuts), some greens, and exudates (gum, nectar).

Herbivores, on the other hand, are "green matter eaters," and are able to break down the cellulose in plant cell walls with the aid of symbiotic microorganisms. They eat mainly vegetative parts of plants (leaves, stems, and roots), which, for humans, would not be considered a primary source of fuel because of their relative indigestibility. Vegetation is rather considered dietary fiber—essential for our health, in part because of our long digestive tracts, but not ideal. The most important realization here is this: organisms need their primary source of fuel to be *wholly* digestible (as fruits are to humans) in order to garner the most amount of nutrients and, therefore, energy. This is a key part of the reason why I am forwarding the argument that humans are naturally frugivores; our bodies are designed to digest fruits and seeds completely, as a primary source of nutrients and fuel, and not stems, roots, and leaves, which are the almost exclusive diet of herbivores.

Secondary Consumer Organisms

Carnivores

Carnivores such as owls, vultures, wolves, and bobcats are called secondary consumer organisms because they derive their energy from eating the flesh of herbivores.

Mixed Consumer Organisms

Omnivores

Omnivores such as opossums, pigs, bears, chickens, emus, and a variety of birds eat plant foods, seeds, and meat for their nourishment and are, therefore, mixed consumer organisms.

Reducer Organisms

Microorganisms

Microbes such as bacteria, fungi, yeast, parasites, and algae are called reducer organisms because their inherent function is to scavenge, decompose, and devour all that is dead and dying back into the dust of the earth, thus cleaning up the environment. Often perceived as pests or germs, reducer organisms are a misunderstood part of the food chain. They are, in essence, nature's clean-up crew—the greatest recyclers ever created. These "germs" are not our enemy and, in truth, we could not live without them!

It was when I began to explore nature's food chain that I began to understand how vitally important *natural feeding* truly is—not just for other living organisms, but for us, too.

EAT RIGHT FOR YOUR ANATOMICAL TYPE

For every type of organism, there is a natural way to feed. As you will see, humans are not designed to be either carnivores or omnivores. Instead, we are intended to be primarily frugivorous. Several hundred years ago, Carolus Linnaeus, the great taxonomist who established scientific methods for classifying plants and animals, recognized that humans were fruit eaters.

> *Man's structure, internal and external compared with*
> *that of the other animals, shows that fruit and*
> *succulent vegetables are his natural food.*
>
> —Carolus Linnaeus (1707-1778)

There may be some who think that eating from the top of the food chain, as the dominant species of omnivore, is more suited to the superior stance of humanity. Some feel it is in our nature to strive to conquer the greatest of beasts. The mightiest of beasts and the most worthy game are carnivores, and when we conquer them, we show ourselves worthy adversaries in a battle to death with the most vicious of foes. We belong in their company. We feed on their flesh and the flesh of all species beneath them in celebration of our dominance, convincing ourselves it is to sustain ourselves and our species. However, natural eating is not about dominating all other life through our mouths. Rather, it is about recognizing our perfect, God-given place within nature. We hold a unique place. We are frugivores—primary consumers—but no species' natural prey. No one hunts us. There are none above us in the food chain.

Francis Moore Lappé, a pioneer in identifying the environmental costs of the foods we eat, suggests that the meat-centered diet is unnatural to humankind. She said:

> Traditionally the human diet has centered on plant foods, with animal foods playing a supplementary role. Our digestive and metabolic system evolved over millions of years on such a diet. Only very recently have Americans, and people in some other industrial countries, begun to center their diets on meat. So it is the meat-centered diet—and certainly the grain-fed-meat-centered diet—that is the fad.

There are many who agree with her. Cardiologist William C. Roberts, MD, hails from the famed cattle state of Texas. He unequivocally believes that humans are not physiologically designed to eat meat, that when we kill animals to eat them, they end up killing us, because their flesh, which contains cholesterol and saturated fat, was never intended for human consumption.

Dr. Roberts says, "I think the evidence is pretty clear. If you look at various physical characteristics of carnivores versus herbivores, it doesn't take a genius to see where humans line up." While Dr. Roberts does not speak to the sub-classes of herbivores, his statement is obvious: humans are not designed to consume meat.

Robert Morse, ND, author of *The Detox Miracle Sourcebook* and "one of the greatest healers of our time" according to Dr. Bernard Jensen—a leading natural health practitioner, and expert in juice therapy, who healed himself from cancer—agrees with Dr. Roberts, except to clarify that humans are not just herbivorous plant eaters, but specifically frugivores because of anatomical design.

To illustrate the feeding habits natural to our anatomical design, Dr. Morse created the following chart comparing the typical anatomy and physiology of carnivores, omnivores, herbivores, and frugivores.

Anatomical Types

Carnivores such as cats, cheetahs, lions	Omnivores such as chickens, pigs, and dogs	Herbivores such as horses, cows, sheep, deer	Primate Frugivores such as humans, apes, chimpanzees, and monkeys
Diet	**Diet**	**Diet**	**Diet**
Mainly meats, some vegetables, grass, and herbs	Some vegetables, meat, fruits, roots, and some barks	Leaves (foliage), herbs, some roots, and barks	Mainly fruits, nuts, sweet vegetables, seeds, and herbs
Digestive system	**Digestive system**	**Digestive system**	**Digestive system**
Very rough tongue (for pulling and tearing)	Moderate to rough tongue	Moderately rough tongue	Smooth tongue, used mainly as a shovel

Carnivores	Omnivores	Herbivores	Primate Frugivores
Digestive system	**Digestive system**	**Digestive system**	**Digestive system**
No salivary glands	Under-active salivary glands	Alkaline digestion starts with the salivary glands	Alkaline digestive energies start with the salivary glands
Stomach has a simple structure; small round sacks; strong gastric juices	Stomach has moderate gastric acids (HCL and pepsin)	Stomach is oblong, ringed, and the most complex (may have 4 or more pouches)	Stomach is oblong with 2 compartments
Small intestine is smooth and short	Small intestine is somewhat sacculated, enabling to eat vegetables	Small intestine is long and sacculated for extensive absorption	Small intestine is sacculated for extensive absorption
Liver is 50% larger than that of humans; very complex with five distinct chambers; heavy bile flow for heavy gastric juices	Liver is complex and larger proportionately than that of humans	Liver is similar to human, though slightly larger in capacity	Liver is simple and average size, not large and complex like carnivores
Eliminative system	**Eliminative system**	**Eliminative system**	**Eliminative system**
Colon is smooth, non-sacculated, with minimal ability for absorption	Colon is shorter than human colon, with minimal absorption	Colon is long and sacculated (ringed) for extensive absorption	Colon is sacculated for extensive absorption
GI tract is 3 times the length of the spine	GI tract is 10 times the length of the spine	GI tract is 30 times the length of the spine	GI tract is 12 times the length of the spine
Extremities	**Extremities**	**Extremities**	**Extremities**
Hands (upper front) with claws	Hands (upper front) are hoofs, claws, or paws	Hands (upper) are hoofs	Hands have fingers for picking, peeling and tearing
Feet (lower back) with claws	Feet (lower back) are hoofs, claws, or paws	Feet (lower) are hoofs	Feet have toes

Carnivores	Omnivores	Herbivores	Primate Frugivores
Quadrupeds (walks on all fours)	Quadrupeds, except for birds, which walk on two legs	Quadrupeds	Walks upright on two feet
Integumentary system	**Integumentary system**	**Integumentary system**	**Integumentary system**
Skin is 100% covered with hair	Skin is smooth, oily, and covered with hair or feathers	Skin has pores with hair covering the whole body	Skin has pores with hair covering the whole body, humans very fine & unnoticeable, others noticeable
Uses tongue to sweat, has sweat glands only in foot pads	Very minimal sweat glands; around snout (pigs) and (foot pads (dogs); none on birds	Millions of perspiration ducts for sweat glands	Millions of perspiration ducts for sweat glands
Skeletal system	**Skeletal system**	**Skeletal system**	**Skeletal system**
Incisor teeth in front, molars behind, large canine teeth for ripping	Tusk-like canine teeth or beaks	24 teeth: 5 molars on each side of upper and lower jaw, and 8 incisors (cutting teeth) in the front of the jaw	32 teeth: 4 incisors, 2 cuspids, 4 small molars, and 6 molars (no long canine or tusklike teeth)
Jaws are unidirectional, up-and-down only	Jaws are multidirectional	Jaws are multidirectional, creating a grinding effect	Jaws are multidirectional
Tail	Tail	Tail	Humans and apes, no tail
Urinary system	**Urinary system**	**Urinary system**	**Urinary system**
Kidneys produce acid urine	Kidneys produce acid urine	Kidneys produce alkaline urine	Kidneys produce alkaline urine

From Robert Morse, N.D., The Detox Miracle Sourcebook (Prescott, AZ: Hohm Press, 2004).

In essence, a cow was not designed to eat a fish or a chicken; it was designed to eat grass. Likewise, a human was not designed to eat a cow or grass; we were designed to eat fruit along with leafy greens and a few nuts and seeds.

Unlike a meat-eating species, we lack both the physical characteristics of carnivores and the instinct that drives us to kill animals and devour their raw carcasses. We are physically and psychologically unable to rip animals limb from limb with our teeth.

Dr. Morse tells us, "Eat the foods that are biologically suited for your species!"

As frugivores, if we found ourselves living in a tropical paradise without modern day conveniences, such as electricity, refrigeration, and grocery stores, our natural diet would be essentially the same as that of a chimpanzee. It would consist of fresh, ripe, raw fruits and some tender, leafy green vegetables and shoots, with the inclusion of small amounts of raw nuts and seeds.

After all, we are essentially 98% genetically and anatomically identical to a chimpanzee. From our teeth to our colons, our entire digestive system is structurally and functionally similar to the other primates. Incidentally, primates have different blood types comparable to humans, and none of them eat differently in a natural setting based upon their blood type.

Raw food advocate Victoria Boutenko, who is also an expert on the raw, living food diet thoroughly researched the diets of chimpanzees for her book *Green for Life*. She tells us,

"Chimpanzees are very similar to humans. Scientists at the Chimpanzee and Human Communication Institute at Washington Central University believe that "chimpanzees should be categorized as people."

So consider eating right for your anatomical type. Eat like a primate! Enjoy lots of alkalizing fruits and greens!

Chapter 3

UNNATURAL FEEDING CAUSES ECOLOGICAL BREAKDOWNS

What we have long called disease is nothing more than a series of ecological breakdowns caused by unnatural feeding!

The ecosystems of the earth are much like the ecosystems of our body. Our land has vast tributaries that run through towns and cities. Communities depend upon these bodies of water and their tributaries for supporting life, transporting commodities from one place to another and being a powerful energy source for hydroelectric plants. For communities to thrive, the ecological equilibrium of tributaries is extremely important.

Similarly, our bodies have an intricate circulatory system made up of a complex network of various-sized tributaries that run through our glands and organs called veins, arteries, and capillaries. Much like our planet's tributaries, our internal tributaries are designed to transport essential commodities such as oxygen and vital nutrients from one area of the body to another.

To fully comprehend how unnatural feeding can disturb our earth's and our body's ecological equilibrium to the point of disease and death, let's consider the near death of one of our nation's greatest bodies of water: Lake Erie.

HOW BODIES OF WATER THRIVE OR DIE

Lake Erie, one of the most productive Great Lakes that divide Canada and the United States, was thriving and replete with life until surrounding industries began feeding industrial waste and sewage into it. As a result of these pollutants, Lake Erie contained increased levels of phosphorus and nitrogen, which contributed to *eutrophication*, a process that encourages the development of algae blooms. Dead fish littered the shoreline as a lack of oxygen in the water led to massive fish kills. Episodes like this led to the coining of the phrase "Lake Erie is dead," which started to appear in national publications in the late 1960s.

How did this happen? In short, because of an ecological imbalance. Algae are an inherent aspect of water ecology when in proper balance with other life forms, and it plays an important role in water health. At that time, some of the most devastating, acidifying pollutants pouring into Lake Erie were organic and inorganic salts of phosphoric acid, commonly called phosphates. Phosphates are food for algae. Unfortunately, algae also require oxygen for their growth process, which they take from the water. So, as the phosphates flooded into the lake, the algae proliferated, doing their job of transforming the abundant supply of acidic chemicals into plant material. At the same time, however, they were using up the precious oxygen in the water faster than it could be replenished. The fish became oxygen-starved and infected with pathogenic bacteria (reducer organisms), and began to die.

Compounding this ecological disaster, Lake Erie's waters became so polluted with oil and petroleum-based sludge, and the gaseous products of rot and fermentation, that the surface of the lake actually caught fire. Fortunately, after the EPA forced shoreline industrial and sewage plants to reduce the dumping frenzy by 80%, the lake, over time, was restored.

At least we thought so.

An article in the *Columbus Dispatch* on November 25, 2012, reports that once again, "Lake Erie is under attack. Toxic algae blooms cover its surface; "dead zones" where fish cannot survive grow beneath the waves; and invasive species crowd out its native plants, fish and mussels." There is recognition that once again, synthetic fertilizer runoffs, particularly the phosphates, are the core issue.

By this time, Lake Erie may be low or depleted of alkalizing minerals like calcium and magnesium. Toxic forms of algae have become entrenched. You could say the Lake has developed a heightened sensitivity to phosphate fertilizer—food that is unnatural to the ecology of a lake.

HOW WE THRIVE OR DIE

Lake Erie's fate is a perfect analogy for understanding how the human body thrives or how it becomes diseased and dies. Like the trillions of fish that swim in the waters of our planet, we too have trillions of cells and vast populations of microorganisms that live throughout the waters of our body. At the microscopic level, our body is mostly cells connected by massive networks of transport passages such as blood vessels. Every organ, every gland, our bones, our skin, our tissues, everything is made up of cells. For our bodies to thrive, ecological equilibrium is absolutely everything!

> *To thrive, cells must live in clean, alkaline water replete with oxygen!*

Unfortunately, most of us are randomly—and even continuously—feeding toxic, acidifying chemicals into our body's systems every day through all of the processed foods we eat, disturbing the ecological equilibrium of our internal environment.

Interestingly, some of the most pervasive acidifying chemicals in the American diet are organic and inorganic phosphates. Organic phosphates are mainly found in meat, eggs, dairy products, grains, legumes, and nuts. Inorganic phosphate additives are found at very high levels in sodas, baked goods, frozen dinners, processed meats, and junk foods of every kind. The inorganic forms of phosphate are even more deadly.

As an internal environmentalist, I have come to the conclusion that the feeding of excessive phosphates into our internal transport passages affects us much as it did Lake Erie. After all, candida (a type of fungus commonly known as yeast) a unicellular organism similar to algae, lives in small colonies throughout our internal environment and is a necessary part of our organism, in balance.

In doing its job to maintain ecological equilibrium, candida, like algae, will overgrow whenever there is excessive food to feed on, or when there is a need to clean up a toxic threat. In the process of proliferating, it too robs the body's cells of precious oxygen, setting the stage for cell death which leads to the breakdown of body systems. If the entire body is threatened by candida, the unicellular organism can morph into a more aggressive, multi-cellular form, which sets the stage for what we call *dis-ease*.

> *Dis-ease: Dis is away from; Ease is a state of being comfortable*

There are numerous symptoms related to candida overgrowth: fatigue, brain fog, depression, low libido, cravings for sugar and alcohol, bloating, food sensitivities, chronic body aches and joint pain, and premature aging are just some. (See more on p. 30.) To compound this already massive ecological disaster, our own internal passageways, like Lake Erie, can become even more polluted. If you consider the additional internal pollution caused by the consumption of animal fats, and processed vegetable fats and oils, which are known promoters of *inflammation*, you can see how our bodies can become even sicker like the near-dead Lake Erie, and full of fire (inflammation).

In essence, what we have long called disease is nothing more than a series of ecological breakdowns caused by unnatural feeding! Moreover, by the time most of us recognize that we have a disease, or are diagnosed, we are well into an acidic, imbalanced state. Some people—those who perish from a heart attack or stroke, for example—never have the opportunity to correct their situation. This perhaps, is, the most frightening aspect of disease, but it can also serve as the motivational reminder that we all need, and must heed, to overcome our current situation.

CANDIDA: THE SILENT KILLER

In its helpful form, *Candida albicans* is a unicellular yeast that naturally lives within our internal environment, such as our blood, lymph, and gastrointestinal tract. The purpose of candida is to assist our inner microbial world in maintaining ecological equilibrium; it is a part of nature's food chain that shows up on the scene whenever there's an impending toxic threat. They are simply nature's "clean-up crew!" As I mentioned above, if the toxic load becomes too extensive, candida is forced to overgrow and even morph into a more aggressive multi-cellular fungal form.

There are several reasons that candida grows out of control:

1. Unnatural feeding; that is, eating a diet high in acidic foods such as meat, dairy, and processed foods loaded with toxic chemicals.
2. Drinking highly acidic drinks, such as sodas and sports drinks.
3. Overeating.
4. A low-oxygen state in the body.

5. Taking drugs such as antibiotics and birth control pills, which destroys the ecological equilibrium of our inner microbial world.
6. Stress, trauma, and emotional upsets.
7. The inability to efficiently eliminate toxic waste.

Left unchecked, the fungus that was meant to be migratory grows into plant-like structures complete with roots. These roots can break through the lining of the gastrointestinal wall, breaking down the protective barrier between the intestinal tract and bloodstream. As a result, proteins and other food wastes that are not completely digested or eliminated can assault the immune system and cause tremendous fatigue, allergic reactions, and numerous other health problems.

This abnormal growth process also allows yeast to travel to other areas of the body, gaining footholds in places where it was never meant to be, creating further complications.

The primary byproduct of candida overgrowth is acetaldehyde, which is converted by the liver into ethanol (alcohol). Ethanol can cause excessive fatigue and a reduction of strength and stamina, which takes away a person's ambition. It destroys enzymes needed for cell energy and causes the release of *free radicals*, which accelerate the aging process.

Here is how to think of free radicals:

> When we think about pH, we usually think of it in terms of the measurement of acidity or alkalinity in a fluid. However, the measurement of pH is really a measurement of voltage, or electrical potential. The greater the electrical potential, the more electrons, and the greater the alkalinity. The less the electrical potential, the fewer the electrons, and the greater the acidity. In a solution of water or tissue, one can have an excess or deficiency of electrons. According to Jerry Tennant, M.D., an excess of electrons is called an "electron donor" and is labeled as negative or alkaline. A deficiency of electrons is called an "electron stealer" and is labeled as positive or acid. Electron stealers cause havoc in the body; they are called *free radicals!* So, if you want to reduce harmful free radicals, *alkalize!*

While it generally goes undiagnosed, candida overgrowth (medically called *candidiasis*) is a silent killer—an incredible destroyer of health, and the missing link in the understanding of our modern diseases. But to believe that candida is the cause of disease is like saying that "roaches cause a dirty kitchen!"

In short, candida is a reducer organism—a part of nature's clean-up crew. So, giving candida a place to blossom and grow by putting the body in an unhealthy state will cause candida to reproduce to unhealthy levels. If you feed 'em, they will come!

Candida-Related Symptoms and Diseases

Candida infections can cause many different symptoms and diseases depending on where in your body the candida overgrowth has colonized. If you are experiencing even a few of these symptoms, you may have candida overgrowth. If you have many of the symptoms listed below, you can rest assured that candida has been in your body a very long time and has most likely spread throughout your internal environment.

Candida Infection Symptoms and Diseases:

Allergies	Diabetes	Low Immunity
Autism	Eczema	Low Sex Drive
Autoimmune Disorders	Fatigue	Low Thyroid
Bad Breath	Fibromyalgia	Migraine Headaches
Brain Fog	Hair Loss	Oral Thrush
Cancer	Headaches	Rashes
Celiac	Intestinal Problems	Sinus, Ear or Eye Infections
Chronic Fatigue	Irritable Bowel	Skin Fungus
Chronic Irritation	Syndrome (IBS)	Toenail Fungus
Chronic Sinusitis	Itchy Red Eyes	Vaginal Yeast Infections
Depression	Jock Itch	Vision Problems
Dermatitis	Joint Pain	Weight Gain
	Low Adrenals	

If you have just one or two of the symptoms shown, and you are not sure whether you have candida overgrowth, this simple candida test may help you to confirm your suspicions, one way or the other.

Candida Test

In the evening, put a clear glass of water by your bed. First thing in the morning, before you put anything into your mouth, work up some saliva and spit it into the glass of water. Keep an eye on the water for half an hour—especially the first few minutes. If you have candida overgrowth, you will see one or more of the following:

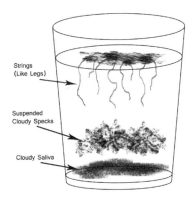

Strings
(Like Legs)

Suspended
Cloudy Specks

Cloudy Saliva

1. Strings (legs) hanging down from the saliva.
2. Heavy-looking saliva at the bottom of the glass.
3. Cloudy specks suspended in the water.

If, within three minutes after spitting into the water, you see "strings" hanging down, cloudy specks showing up in the water, or globs of spit sinking to the bottom, you most likely have extensive overgrowth. If it takes longer than a few minutes for anything to show up, the candida is not as serious. If the saliva just floats on top and the water stays perfectly clear, you most likely don not have candida overgrowth. In essence, the more you see, and the sooner you see it, the more systemic the infection.

How Does The Candida Test Work?

The logic behind the Candida Spit Test is simple. Candida overgrowth begins in the colon. Over time, as the fungal yeast multiplies it begins to migrate through the digestive tract, moving up into the small intestine, then the stomach (bloating, indigestion), up the esophagus and into the mouth. If it becomes strongly entrenched there, you can see a white film on your tongue and inside your cheeks. Once it has moved up to the mouth, when you spit into a glass of water the yeast will sink, because it is denser than water. If there is no yeast, it will float on top.

An overgrowth of candida is an S-O-S signal warning you that your body is susceptible to diabetes and various other diseases such as cancer.

DIABETES: THE CAUSE, THE CURE

Up until now, we have believed that eating too much sugar—even natural sugar found in fruit—is what causes Type 2 diabetes. However, this may not be the whole picture. Let's consider what happens to the cells when they become infected with oxygen-robbing candida.

According to Dr. Graham, author of *The 80/10/10 Diet*, candida is a microbe that lives in our intestines, as well as other tissues in the body, and our bloodstream, and is regulated by blood sugar and friendly bacteria. In fact, candida is a food source for the friendly and protective bacteria in our body called "acidophillus and bifidus." It is inherently designed to be there, in moderate amounts, as previously mentioned.

Candida's food is blood sugar, and when our blood sugar is present in normal amounts the amount of candida remains stable and our internal environment thrives.

The problem arises when blood sugar becomes excessive and candida is forced to multiply to eliminate the toxic threat of excessive sugar. Insulin is the hormone that delivers glucose into the cell. Glucose is a simple sugar that is an extremely important energy source for our body. If a person's insulin is unable to do its job of escorting glucose to the cell because there's too much sugar in the blood for the insulin to handle, candida keeps blooming. What inhibits insulin from escorting glucose into the cells for energy production is the overconsumption of extracted fats. Fats clog the cell membranes, preventing the transference of glucose. The more fat in your diet, the less effective insulin is at getting glucose into the cells and out of the bloodstream. When there is excessive glucose in the bloodstream, there is Type 2 diabetes. This is why Type 2 diabetes is 100% reversible through a proper (low-fat) diet, and exercise; the body's normal glucose transfer can be restored when fats are burned and reduced. As a side note, while the majority of people who develop Type 2 diabetes are overweight, some are thin. The cause of the problem, however, is the same.

Unlike the traditional anti-candida diet of no fruit and low carbohydrates, Dr. Graham concluded that a high fruit diet, with a very small amount of fat, will not only stop the overgrowth of candida, but over time, it will reverse most every symptom known.

> Candida is similar to algae. It is a microorganism that naturally lives in our body's tissues and bloodstream. Its food is blood sugar! The unnatural feeding of too much fat is what causes it to grow out of control.

This sentiment is echoed by Neal Barnard, MD, author of *Neal Barnard's Program for Reversing Diabetes*, who suggests that people with Type 2 diabetes, or those at risk for diabetes, accumulate abnormal fat droplets inside muscle and liver cells, which leads to insulin resistance.

Insulin resistance, as we described above, is the first stage of Type 2 diabetes. It occurs because the cells (like the fish that are forced to swim in an oil spill) have become clogged with oil. When cell membranes become clogged with fat, insulin—the hormone that escorts glucose into the cells—is unable to do its job, so glucose builds up in the bloodstream.

They call this diabetes; I call it an *ecological breakdown!*

Dr. Barnard's research showed that minimizing dietary fat, especially animal fat found in meat, eggs, and dairy, directly reduces or eliminates the fat deposits in muscle cells. He also found that the same holds true with extracted vegetable oils. While animal fat is the big villain, most vegetable oils, which are 100% extracted fats, should be eliminated as well.

Dr. Barnard concluded that a high-fiber, naturally low-fat, plant-based, vegan diet reduces insulin resistance, improves insulin sensitivity, and reduces elevated glucose levels in the blood. These are signs of a restored cellular environment.

CANCER: THE CAUSE, THE CURE

"Breast cancer is an environmental disease that has to do with the fats and synthetic chemicals in your diet."

—John McDougall, MD, author of *The McDougall Plan: 12 Days to Dynamic Health*

Up until now, we have called one of our nation's most feared diseases—cancer—a mystery. But what if there is a tie-in between the overconsumption of fat, excessive sugar in the bloodstream, acidosis (too much acid in the body's tissues), low oxygen levels, candida overgrowth, and cancer?

Let's take a look.

The cause of cancer is no longer a mystery—cancer is a fungus!

—Dr. Tullio Simoncini

In his book *Cancer Is a Fungus*, Italian oncologist Tullio Simoncini reveals his discovery that cancer does not depend on mysterious causes of genetic, immunological or auto-immunological origin. Instead, it develops from a simple fungal infection, which is always present in the tissues of cancer patients, especially in terminal patients.

For about 100 years, the medical theory behind cancer has been based on the hypothesis that it is a malfunctioning of the genes. This point of view implies that cancer is *intracellular* (from within the cell). Dr. Simoncini's point of view, however, is that cancer is a fungal infection, and therefore an *extracellular* (from outside of the cell) phenomenon. Dr. Simoncini is encouraging modern oncology researchers, who spend millions upon millions of dollars each year on studies that yield only minimally useful results, to move cancer research into the study of microorganisms in an attempt to solve the mysteries of cancer once and for all.

However, as it would be unwise to blame the death of Lake Erie on the overgrowth of algae, it would be similarly unwise to blame cancer on candida. I believe that fungus is *not* the cause of cancer, but that the cause is an acidic, low oxygen environment created by the out-of-control proliferation of anaerobic fungus (candida). In other words, cancer develops and thrives by the proliferation of fungus within the tissues and fluids of a *low-oxygenated body*. Thus, it is the environment that creates the conditions for cancer to exist.

They may call this cancer, but I call it an *ecological breakdown!*

As far back as 1924, Dr. Otto Warburg, who was twice a Nobel laureate, reported that the primary *cause* of cancer is the replacement of aerobic respiration (the inhalation and exhalation of oxygen) in normal body cells by anaerobic respiration (the conversion of food to energy without oxygen).

Dr. Warburg firmly believed that *fermentation,* the anaerobic conversion of sugar to carbon dioxide and alcohol by yeast, is the metabolic pathway of cancer cells, mostly due to his discovery of its association with low oxygen levels, lactic acid production (a by-product of fermentation), and elevated carbon dioxide (CO_2) levels. Yeast cells give off CO2 in their respiration whereas normal cells give off oxygen in their respiration.

Dr. Warburg demonstrated that all forms of cancer are characterized by two basic conditions: *acidosis* (too much acid in the body's tissues), and low oxygen levels. He reported that acidosis and low oxygen levels are two sides of the same coin: where you have one you have the other.

In his later years, Dr. Warburg was so convinced that disease resulted from acidosis and low oxygen levels that, even though his colleagues deemed him a "health nut," he would eat only organically grown fruits and vegetables. The link between an acidic environment, caused by eating acidic foods, cellular oxygen deprivation, and disease had been firmly established in his mind, and he altered his own way of life as a result. Evidence of the connection between an acidic diet and disease dates back nearly a century.

More recent research by Dr. Stephen Levine, molecular biologist and geneticist, and Paris Kidd, PhD (speciality in Antioxidant Adaptation) indicates the likelihood that the switch from aerobic to anaerobic respiration in the cell is mediated by free radical damage. As the structure of the suffocating cell comes under attack from free radicals and internal communication is impaired, the proliferating fungus takes over the function of energy production through fermentation.

Under normal conditions, a deeply damaged cell triggers its own death (called apoptosis)—a sacrifice to protect the larger community of the body. In saving the damaged cell, the fungus creates a monster—a monster we call cancer.

Here are what two other highly acclaimed medical experts have to say about the health hazards of an acidic, oxygen-deprived environment.

- Noted German scientist and microbiologist Dr. Gunther Enderlein (1872–1968), stated, "Basically, there is not a multitude of diseases, but only one constitutional disease, namely the constant over-acidification of the blood…all of which is mainly the result of an inverted way of living and eating."

- Ed McCabe, MD, and author of *Flood Your Body with Oxygen: Therapy for Our Polluted World*, says, "The bacteria, the viruses, the cancer cells, the fungus, the pathogens, almost all these microbes are anaerobic. Anaerobic is the scientific term that means they can't live in oxygen. So I discovered over a hundred years' worth of research, actual medical history, going back documenting doctors that were using different oxygen therapies and products [to reverse these low-oxygen conditions]."

Viewing our modern day diseases through the eyes of an internal environmentalist has shifted everything for me. I now believe that cancer, like diabetes and other degenerative diseases, progresses through a series of ecological breakdowns.

Here's and overview of how I believe it happens:

- When we feed on acidic foods and extracted oils, the passageways that our cells are swimming in become acidic, low in oxygen, and polluted with fungus, and rancid, oily sludge (undigested food particles).

- Our cells become clogged, literally gasping for oxygen like fish in a lake overgrown with algae or that become saturated in oil and die when there is an oil spill.

- Sugar builds up in the bloodstream, due to the fact that its carrier, insulin, is unable to penetrate the cell wall to supply fuel for energy production.

- Candida and other species of fungus grow out of control as they feed on blood sugar.

- If left unchecked, over time the fluids of our body can become so inflamed and overrun with fungus that anaerobic fermentation sets in.
- The suffocating, crumbling cells, no longer able to control their own functions, are taken over and switched from aerobic respiration to anaerobic fermentation under the new domain of a fungal infestation.

- A cancer/fungal cell forms and, if left unchecked, the four stages of cancer ensue.

From this standpoint, the cause and cure of most known diseases hinge on the types of food we feed into our internal environment: acid or alkaline, processed or whole. Acid foods such as meat, dairy, and processed foods loaded with toxic chemicals create an acidic, low-oxygen environment. Alkaline foods such as fruits and vegetables create an alkaline, oxygen-rich environment. Acid foods are the cause—alkaline foods are the cure.

To turn any internal environmental crisis around that you may be faced with, keep in mind that unnatural feeding is what spawns our inner world of microbes to produce life and health, death or disease. The condition of your environment is everything.

You are alkaline by design, and an alkaline environment replete with oxygen is a place where health thrives and disease cannot exist.

Chapter 4

THE INTERNAL
ACID RAIN THEORY

*Is acid rain running through your veins, destroying your
inner rainforest, depleting most of your life-giving oxygen?*

Let's consider another way ecosystems disintegrate and die: acid rain. Because of the reduction in power plant emissions, which have reduced acid rain in some parts of the world, we don't hear much about acid rain these days. But it is still a serious issue.

Like the ecosystems of the human body, the planet's soils and rivers have alkaline reserves that neutralize the effects of acid rain. Let's see what happens when those reserves are depleted.

HOW ACID RAIN DESTROYS OUR PLANET

Acid rain forms in our planet's environment when toxic wastes and by-products are released into the atmosphere from certain industrial and agricultural practices, as well as from the burning of fossil fuels such as natural gas, coal, and oil. These pollutants react in the atmosphere with water, oxygen, and other chemicals and form various compounds, resulting in an acidic residue or "ash" that can be carried through the atmosphere for hundreds of miles from its origin. As moisture condenses around the acidic ash, these compounds return to the earth by way of rain, snow, or fog. The effect is acid rain—a condensation that is defined as having a pH level of 5.5 or below.

To the naked eye, acid rain does not look any different from normal rain, but don't be fooled. Acid rain destroys everything it touches. Bodies of water, soils, and plant life are profoundly affected by acidic rainfall as illustrated in the drawing below.

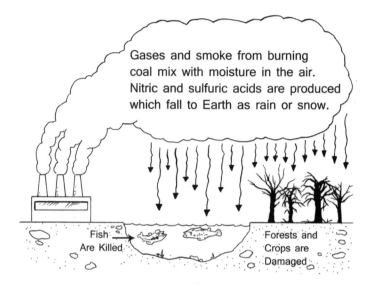

How Acid Rain Destroys Aquatic Ecosystems

Earth's unpolluted waters have a natural alkaline pH value that ranges between 7 and 8. The flora and fauna that swim in these bodies of water thrive in their naturally alkaline environment; they die in an acidic environment. Sadly, when acid rain falls directly into Earth's tributaries or washes into them as surface runoff, the naturally alkaline environment is greatly altered, becoming more acidic.

Some bodies of water have sub-aquatic soils and bedrock capable of buffering increased acidity; others do not. Buffering capacity—the ability to neutralize fluctuations in acidity or alkalinity—is based on mineral content. A low mineral content equates to a weak buffering capacity. When the buffering capacity is low, and the acid-rain onslaught is high, heavy metals such as aluminum, which are normally bound to soil and bedrock, are released and they poison aquatic life.

Once the readily available "alkaline reserves" of soils or riverbeds are depleted, these ecosystems become ever more vulnerable to the debilitating effects of acid rain. One mitigation technique involves lining a river with limestone. The limestone provides a new reserve of alkalizing minerals to combat both acidity and toxic levels of aluminum that were activated by acid rain.

The oceans also contain alkalizing minerals like lime (calcium carbonate). This gives them a strong buffering capacity. This is a critical function because even a small change in the pH of the ocean can have devastating effects on life—sea life for sure, but also land inhabitants like humans. Many species rely on a consistently alkaline environment to survive. When that environment acidifies, their lives are threatened. With even a small movement toward acidification, dissolved oxygen can disappear, as is happening in many oceanic dead zones around the world. Dead zones are what they sound like: places where life no longer exists.

How Acid Rain Destroys Rainforest Ecosystems

Acid rain destroys rainforest ecosystems, such as soil and trees. Green plants and the soil they inhabit are essential to life on our planet. Plants fill our atmosphere with lots of oxygen. Without them, life as we know it would not exist.

Consider that a tree has a trunk, branches, and foliage, which are insulated with a waxy protective coating essential to the tree's immunity from harsh weather, parasites, and disease. But when acid rain falls onto a tree, it eats away at its waxy protective coating, exposing the tree's previously protected foliage and limbs to the elements, and creating a breakdown called oxidation—a process that destroys the structural integrity of the tree. This is when the tree's immunity begins to be compromised.

Also consider that a tree has a root system that has tiny hairs, which are responsible for extracting, absorbing, and transferring nutrients into the tree. Mostly unseen by the human eye, there are billions of microorganisms that inhabit the upper layers of the soil. These microorganisms break down mineral and dead organic matter into compounds that provide the nutrients necessary for plant growth. When acid rain falls onto the earth, it not only destroys the host of living microorganisms within the upper layers of the soil, it also depletes the nutrients from the soil, causing a decline in plant growth and further weakening of the immunity of the tree.

Heavy metals such as aluminum, mercury, and cadmium, which are normally bound to minerals, are released by the acidic condition of the soil and are absorbed through the tiny hairs of the tree's root system. As the toxic metals continue to build up, they block the flow of vital nutrients, poison the tree, further weakening its immunity. Over time, the tree's root system weakens and breaks down, which causes decaying matter to build up inside the root. The tree completely loses its immunity as it begins to rot and decay. The tree becomes susceptible to insects, disease, drought, and severe weather.

Reducer organisms like bacteria, yeast, fungus, and mold, previously held in check by the immunity of the tree, arrive on the scene to convert what is dead and dying back into the dust of the earth. Eventually, the tree falls to the earth and is completely absorbed by the soil.

So, instead of using toxic pesticides to kill the bugs we call the enemy, perhaps we should ask: *Why have these bugs arrived on the scene?*

HOW INTERNAL ACID "RAIN" DESTROYS OUR BODY

Food is broken down in the digestive tract and used as fuel through various metabolic processes. One of those processes is called *oxidation,* a chemical reaction whereby oxygen binds itself to an element or compound and then is essentially "burned" by the body for fuel. What is not used for fuel is a residue known as *ash.* This is a similar process to burning wood in a stove, whereby oxygen unites with the wood to produce carbon dioxide and water vapor that passes up through the chimney as smoke; the ashes remain in the stove.

This ash, depending on what types of foods are consumed, can be either acid or alkaline. Thus, we can divide *fuel foods* into two distinctive categories: acid and alkaline ash–forming foods.

When acid ash–forming foods are eaten, internal acidity—we might say an internal acid rain—is formed as bodily fluids condense around the acid ash that is left from the "burn." This condensation can have a pH level of 5.5 or even lower. The acid ash then travels throughout our body's internal tributaries, depositing its destructive ash throughout our body—just like acid rain deposits its destructive ash on our earth.

How Internal Acid Rain Destroys Our Body's Aquatic Ecosystems

Our earth's massive network of oceans has currents that move its waters long distances and between deep and shallow waters.

Like the earth, our body also has an aquatic ecosystem: our circulatory system. The circulatory system consists of two types of fluids: blood and lymph. These fluids are responsible for carrying nutrients to and from every organ and gland, along with the trillions of cells that live within these fluids.

Now let's take a look at how high acidity destroys our body's aquatic ecosystems. Sadly, when acid ash inhabits our internal "tributaries," our natural alkaline pH is altered, which results in lower oxygen levels in our blood and lymph. Even a small change in the pH of the bloodstream can tip us toward acidosis, disease and death.

Like the earth's buffering system (described previously), we, too, have the ability to neutralize either overly acidic or overly alkaline states. The body's capacity to buffer acids is based on the quantity of alkalizing minerals in our fluids and bones. When we are low on alkalizing minerals, we have a weak capacity to buffer the acid ash floating around in fluids and tissues. When our buffering capacity is weak, and the acid onslaught great, in part from a diet high in meat and other animal products, heavy metals such as aluminum, which are normally bound to our bones and tissue, are released and further poison our cells. The acid within us does to our bodies exactly what acid rain does to the planet—it destroys everything in its path.

How Internal Acid Rain Destroys Our Body's Ecosystems

Like the trees of the earth, we, too, suffer the consequences of a highly acidic environment—as trees suffer from acid rain, we suffer from our own acidic internal fluids. As a tree has bark as an outer covering, we have skin. As a tree has a trunk, we have a torso, which houses our spinal column, the body's "tree of life." Just as the tree's branches have a waxy protective covering that shields them from the elements, our nerves have a fatty protective coating, which also shields them from external threat. This waxy protective coating around our nerves is known as the *myelin sheath.* In the same manner that acid rain strips the waxy protective coating on the foliage of a tree, internal acids can also strip the myelin sheath from around our nerves.

Our intestinal tract is a bit like the root system of a tree. Instead of the fine hairs on the outside of a root, however, our intestines have fine hairs on the inside, called *villi.*

Villi, like the fine hairs on a tree's root system, are responsible for extracting, absorbing, and transferring nutrients from one part of the body to another.

There are billions of microorganisms that exist within our intestinal tract, just like there are in the soil of the earth, surrounding a tree's roots. The job of our own microorganisms is to break down food and beverages into absorbable nutrients. Sadly, these beneficial microorganisms are destroyed from the onslaught of high internal acid levels—in the same way a tree's soils suffer from acid rain.

Our intestinal ecosystem is further destroyed when heavy metals enter the environment of our intestines and plug up our villi, inhibiting the uptake of nutrients and lowering our immunity. So, like the tree, we continue to weaken and lose our vitality, and become susceptible to disease.

Reducer organisms in the form of bacterial, yeast and fungus, which are a necessary part of nature's clean-up crew, arrive on the scene to break down what is dead and dying and convert it back into the dust of the earth.

VALIDATION OF THE INTERNAL ACID RAIN THEORY

To validate the *internal acid rain theory*, Lorne Label, MD conducted pH studies on some of his patients who had been stricken with neurological diseases. We had discussed the latest medical research that revealed *Chlamydia* bacteria could be the cause of these devastating diseases. They were almost always present in those suffering from Parkinson's, Alzheimer's, and multiple sclerosis.

Agreeing with me that bacteria were opportunistic, and most likely not the originating cause of these diseases, he decided to perform a number of spinal taps on some of his patients to test the pH of their cerebrospinal fluid.

About a month later, Dr. Label reported back.

> After contemplating your internal acid rain theory, I performed a number of spinal taps on Alzheimer's, Parkinson's, and multiple sclerosis patients, as the cerebral spinal fluid is, in effect, the brain's "water" supply and should have a pH value of approximately 7.4. When I tested the cerebrospinal fluid's pH, to my amazement, you were right: it was approximately 5.5—the pH of environmental

acid rain. Further dietary research is justified to see if shifting the pH of the brain terrain will provide clues in turning these devastating diseases around. From the evidence I now see, I am optimistic.

So, again, instead of using antibiotics to kill the bugs we call the enemy, perhaps we should ask: Why have these bugs arrived on the scene in the first place? Perhaps, then, we will begin to apply truly effective solutions.

THE FOUR STAGES OF INTERNAL ACID RAIN

Internal acidity—akin to external acid rain—occurs whenever we "burn" (consume and digest) foods that leave an acid ash in our internal environment. Other contributors include unresolved trauma, negative thoughts and emotions, excessive stress, the use of personal care or household cleaning products loaded with toxic chemicals, pharmaceutical and street drugs, smoking, toxic indoor air, lack of exercise or rest, shallow breathing, dehydration, radiation, and lack of sunshine. Any of these conditions generate and accelerate the ecological breakdown of our internal environment.

As I see it, internal acid rain is the root cause of most every degenerative disease and progresses through four distinct stages of ecological breakdown.

STAGE 1
Autointoxication

Autointoxication takes place when we constantly burn acid-ash foods and other acidifying substances for fuel in our internal environment. Over time, as acid ash and polluted waste accumulates, our internal terrain becomes overly acidic; our organs and glands become congested and sluggish and ineffective at performing their jobs.

Some of the physical and emotional conditions associated with this first stage of internal acidity are low energy, mild depression, muscle tension, digestive disorders, headache, sore throat, irritability, skin eruptions, kidney or bladder infection, muscle aches, bloating, anxiety, hypoglycemia, short attention span, hyperactivity, confusion, sinus pressure, mucous drainage, weight gain or loss, nightmares, hypersensitivity or emotional volatility. Over time, if acidic wastes and toxic metals are not properly eliminated, they settle deeper into the tissues, causing a more serious condition to develop depending on the area in which they reside.

STAGE 2
Autoimmunization

Autoimmunization takes place when the immune system begins a self-attacking, misdirected response to the continual accumulation of heavy metals, polluted waste, and acid ash throughout the blood, lymph, and tissues of our body. The immune system becomes so compromised that it is unable to prevent the onslaught of microbial invasions, and the body begins to attack the microorganisms. If this microbial war is not dealt with, an inflammatory response is triggered by the immune system in an attempt to repair the damage.

Chronic symptoms progress toward environmental or food allergies, migraine headaches, high blood pressure, irritable bowel syndrome, leaky gut, acid reflux, celiac disease, Crohn's disease, high cholesterol, asthma, sinus infections, lupus, chronic fatigue syndrome, fibromyalgia, kidney stones, gallstones, Parkinson's, Alzheimer's, multiple sclerosis, bronchial pneumonia, arthritis, depression, obesity, addictions, and diabetes.

STAGE 3
Autoinfection

Autoinfection takes place with the proliferation of microbial organisms in a highly toxic environment. Cell death accelerates and the body is now in a full-blown state of chronic acidosis. Systemic candida infection rages out of control. The body's immunity becomes overwhelmed in its attempt to sustain ecological equilibrium. If the body's SOS signal is not heeded, the automatic immune response is unremitting reinfection with larvae produced by parasites and worms. In essence, the undertakers have arrived on the scene.

Some of the physical conditions associated with this advanced stage of acidification are: heart attack, cancer, AIDS, and advanced expressions of stage-two, autoimmune conditions.

STAGE 4

Auto-Predictable Death!

If you, or someone you love, are presently suffering from any of these progressive stages, maybe you can finally let go of the theory that germs are your enemy and take hold of the truth behind what the philosopher Pogo once said:

We have met the real enemy and the enemy is us!

Chapter 5

HOW TO CONDUCT AN INTERNAL ACID RAIN STUDY

Your urine is your body's rainwater, so test it to see
if acid rain is destroying your inner rainforest.

Fortunately, there's a way for you to see firsthand how an unnatural diet high in acid-ash foods creates an internal acid rain. There's also a way to determine the present condition of your internal environment. By testing your urine and saliva, you can see whether the types of food you've been burning for fuel have compromised your inner rainforest and depleted your life-giving oxygen.

Like environmentalists who conduct acid-rain tests to check the pH levels of the rain falling within geographical regions, you, too, can conduct tests within your own internal environment. I call this the *internal acid rain study.*

Saliva is the entry point of digestion while urine is the final outward flow of elimination. Each tells us different things. Just keep in mind that these pH tests are not meant to be comprehensive diagnostic tools; they are only meant to give you an indication of a potential problem.

ACID AND ALKALINE ASH–FORMING FOODS

Before beginning your environmental study, it is important to review the acid/alkaline food chart below; it will greatly assist you with your food choices while performing the acid rain study. Keep in mind that if a food increases the acidity of urine, it is classified as an acid ash–forming food that is ecologically unfriendly to your internal environment. Conversely, if a food increases the alkalinity of urine, it is classified as an alkaline ash–forming food that is "green," or ecologically friendly to your internal environment.

The following is a summary of which foods are the most and the least acid ash and alkaline ash–forming foods.

Strong Acid Ash–Forming Foods	Mild Acid Ash–Forming Foods
Red meat	Fish
Pork	Grains
Chicken	Beans or Legumes
Eggs	Nuts
Dairy	Seeds
Processed, chemical-laden foods	

Strong Alkaline Ash–Forming Foods	Mild Alkaline Ash–Forming Foods
Wheatgrass	Fruits
Green leafy vegetables	Vegetables
Green juices and powders	Sea vegetables

Note: All organic, unrefined cold-pressed fats and oils have a neutral pH, being neither acid nor alkaline. Nevertheless, foods that have been altered in any way from their whole, natural form, including extracted oils, have an acidifying effect on the body's ecological equilibrium.

OUR BODY'S BUFFERING CAPACITY

An internal acid rain study is all about *buffering capacity*. Buffering capacity refers to the ability of a fluid to maintain a stable pH as acids are added. If a solution has sufficient buffering capacity, it can absorb and neutralize the addition of some acids without a significant change in the pH. In essence, buffering capacity is a measure of resilience.

Conceptually, a buffer acts somewhat like a sponge. As more acid is added, the "sponge" absorbs the acid without much change in the pH. However, the capacity of the buffering sponge is limited. Once the buffering capacity is used up, the pH changes more rapidly as acids continue to be added.

As mentioned earlier, our capacity to buffer acids is mainly dependent upon our *alkaline reserves.* Alkaline reserve refers to stores of alkalizing minerals that are available to neutralize acids. A healthy body generally has a large storehouse of alkaline reserves, a sick body does not.

The body has an innate intelligence, and it knows how and when to draw from our internal reserves and how and when to restore those reserves, especially when we live within the rhythms of nature.

The problem arises when our buffering capacity is constantly called upon to pull minerals from our alkaline reserves. Eventually, we run low, and our body loses its capacity to neutralize acids, which leaves our internal environment in a vulnerable position.

URINE pH TESTS

These urine pH tests will give you information about how acids are being neutralized. You might imagine that if your buffering capacity is superb, a healthy urine test would always be at pH 7, but it is a little more complicated. There are several alkalizing systems at play, and by taking these tests, you will find out how to determine which systems are kicking in and what that means for your internal terrain.

To perform a urine test, you can either use litmus paper or pH sticks, which can be found at most health-food stores. You may even be inspired to enroll your children, family members, or a close friend to take the test with you and compare scores. It is fun, informative, and life changing. Children especially enjoy it.

Today, most schools teach our children about ecosystems and how acid rain affects the environment in which they live. They are taught to do an environmental study by collecting the earth's rainwater, then checking its pH. If the collected rainwater's pH has a measurement of 5.5 or lower, it is defined as an acid rain that is creating damage in the environment.

Yes, your urine is an external gauge of the fuel you have been burning for fuel into your body!

Day 1—Baseline Test

Your urine should always reflect the type of ash you have just burned for fuel. So begin this test before making any changes to your diet. This will give you a baseline reading so that you'll be able to chart your results as change evolves and ecological equilibrium is restored.

Eat the foods you would normally eat for one entire day (24 hours). Before going to bed, place a disposable cup next to your commode. The next morning upon waking, collect your first morning urine. Dip the pH stick into the urine and shake off the excess. Compare the color with the color chart and record your results. Depending on what you ate, your measurement should read between 5.8 and 7.4.

If you ate mostly acid ash–forming foods the previous day, your pH should read between 5.8 and 6.0; the color of the pH paper will be yellow. If you have eaten mostly alkaline ash–forming foods, your pH should read between 6.4 and 6.8; the color of the pH paper will be light green. If you ate all alkaline ash–forming foods, your pH should read between 7.0 and 7.4; the color of the pH paper will be a darker green.

Day 2—Acid Meal Test

Caution: If you are really sick, or have a serious chronic disease, skip this test!

To perform the internal acid rain study, devote one entire day (24 hours) to eating only acid ash–forming foods such as meat, pasta, beans, bread, fish, dairy, and eggs. If you are already a vegetarian or vegan, just eat the foods in your regime that are more acid ash–forming, such as wheat, sugar, and beans. Have no alkaline–forming foods at all—no vegetables, fruits, or their juices.

Upon waking the next morning, repeat the urine test. Your urine should reflect the ash from the foods eaten the day before, which was acid. Thus, a normal pH reading would be approximately 5.5—the pH of acid rain.

Day 3—Alkaline Meal Test

Devote one entire day (24 hours) to eating only alkaline ash–forming foods such as raw fruits and vegetables and their juices. Have no acid ash–forming foods at all: no wheat, sugar, beans, chemicalized processed foods, dairy, meat, coffee, or tea (refer to the acid list given). You will also want to exclude any nutritional supplements you are presently taking. Upon waking the next morning, repeat the urine test. Your urine should reflect the ash from the foods eaten the day before, which is alkaline. Thus, a healthy pH reading would be 7.0 to 7.2.

How to Interpret the Results

Your urine should always reflect the type of ash you have just burned for fuel. Thus, if you eat a diet high in acid ash–forming foods for 24 hours, the ash in your first morning urine should measure 5.5, the pH of acid rain. If it is between 6.0 and 6.6, it is a sure sign that your alkaline reserves are low, and stronger, secondary back-up systems are being called upon to supplement them. A reading between 6.8 and 8.0 means the kidneys are producing ammonia as a last resort to neutralize acids. This is a sign that your alkaline reserves are dangerously low.

On the other hand, after eating only alkaline ash–forming foods for 24 hours, your pH numbers should be approximately 7.2. In this case, if your pH numbers are lower than 7.0, it is a sign that your alkaline reserves are low.

For a more in-depth understanding, I recommend Dr. Ted Morter, Jr.'s books, especially *Correlative Urinalysis and Your Health Your Choice.*

SALIVA PH TEST

The pH of the saliva fluid parallels that of the extracellular fluid. This fluid is the "inner sea" your cells are swimming in, and is the most consistent and definitive way to measure your body's pH levels and buffering capacity. When a person is healthy, the pH of their blood is approximately 7.4, the pH of their spinal fluid is approximately 7.4, and the pH of their first morning saliva is approximately 7.4.

The saliva test measures the pH of your internal tributaries.

The first morning saliva pH of a healthy person should be between 7.2 and 7.4. The lower you go on the pH scale the more acid you are, which means the more deficient you are in alkalizing minerals. A pH range from 7.0 to 6.5 is slightly acid; 6.5 to 5.5 is mildly acid; and 5.5 to 4.5 is severely acid.

According to Robert Barefoot and Carl Reich, authors of *The Calcium Factor: The Scientific Secret of Health and Youth,* most infants have a pH of 7.5 while more than one-half of the adult population has a saliva pH of 6.5 or lower. Cancer patients usually have a saliva pH of 4.5, especially in the advanced stages. Their research shows that virtually all degenerative diseases, including cancer, heart disease, osteoporosis, arthritis, kidney and gall stones, and tooth decay, are associated with excess acidity in the body.

The most accurate way to test your saliva pH is to measure it first thing in the morning, even before drinking water or brushing your teeth. You can also test it at other times, but wait at least 2 hours after drinking or eating. To test, fill your mouth with saliva, stir with your tongue, and then swallow. Do this several times to help ensure that your saliva is clean. Fill your mouth with saliva and put some saliva onto a small strip of pH paper.

When measuring your first morning saliva pH, if your body's tissues and fluids are alkaline and your buffering capacity is high, the pH paper should turn dark green, indicating an overall internal environment pH of approximately 7.2. If it is below 7.0, your tributaries are acid, indicating that your alkaline minerals and oxygen levels are low—the more acid, the greater the depletion. This is a value that does not change much from day to day, that is, until you make a concerted effort to clean up the acids and bring balance back to your internal tributaries.

This brings me to my next point: who is responsible for your health? As you contemplate this question, and consider the role of your doctor regarding the safeguarding of your health, keep in mind these words from Hippocrates—for whom the famed Hippocratic Oath (an oath that most doctors in America to this day elect to take upon graduation) is named:

> The physician must be able to tell the antecedents (ancestors), know the present, and foretell the future. He must mediate these things, and have two special objects in view with regard to disease, namely, to do good or to do no harm.

I've provided some general clues in Part I about how Hippocrates identified the causes of disease and death and, therefore, of health. Within this framework, perhaps you can understand your present condition, and will want to predict (or change!) the future unfolding. This is you becoming responsible for your health, which is a wonderful thing! The key is becoming a student of nature, thus your own physician!

Of course, the choice is yours. You can wait for death to knock at your door—like I did—or you can begin now to cultivate your internal environment so that instead of being a toxic wasteland, your body can become the instrument it was designed to be.

If you are curious, use the simple tests I've given you in the last chapter to get a general picture of the health of your internal environment. If you already know that you are in the midst of an internal environmental crisis, and are ready to turn it around, then keep reading!

In Part II, you are going to find out how to eliminate the foods that no longer serve you and begin the process of creating an internal alkaline environment—the basis for a disease-free life!

When you do, every cell of your body will become like an alkaline battery so you, too, can keep going on…on and on and on!

PART TWO

ECODIET

The Ecotarian Revolution!

Chapter 6

IT'S TIME TO STOP THE DIETARY DEVOLUTION MOVEMENT

*Dietary Devolution is how we are
destroying our bodies and our planet.*

Sad, but true; we have moved far away from a diet that supports our natural, anatomical design—a diet of fruits, leafy greens, shoots, wild vegetation, and occasional nuts and seeds. For most, unnatural feeding has become a habitual way of life. The devolution took place throughout the ages of time as we slowly but surely shifted predominantly from an alkaline fruit- and plant-based diet as *frugivores* to a predominantly acid, animal-based diet as *omnivores*.

In the last century, in particular, *dietary* devolution has slid even further down the scale, from an acidic *omnivore* diet. This is because of the advent of the even more acidic *chemivore* diet, the strongly acidic *junkivore* diet, and the extremely acidic drugivore diet (see my definitions below). These are new terms, admittedly, but they are meant to illustrate a point: not only have we moved far away from our natural diet, but many of us are now consuming "foods" that are not even foods!

The scope of dietary devolution is not only destroying our body's ecosystems but our planet's ecosystems as well. In a very fundamental way, dietary devolution is associated with the belief that we are separate from the earth; it is as if we've forgotten where we have come from, and that the majority of species on this planet subsist on natural foods from the earth. Moreover, we now believe that we can actually create a better form of food in a laboratory. Do you see the madness?

Dietary devolution is characterized by the following:

1. **Omnivore Diet:** The addition of domesticated animal flesh and animal products to the frugivore diet, eventually eclipsing the frugivore diet. The substitution of cooked foods for raw foods and the addition of cultivated grains and beans complete the picture.

2. **Chemivore Diet:** Petro-chemically, radioactively and genetically contaminated plant foods, animal flesh and products.

3. **Junkivore Diet:** Chemivore foods that have been highly processed, denatured, and chemically altered. In some cases, chemical substitutions are made for real food.

4. **Drugivore Diet:** A handful of synthetic drugs for breakfast, lunch, and dinner.

In writing about dietary devolution, I have a twofold intention: to unmask the grave problems we face, and to give you useful knowledge about how to navigate through the modern food system and stop the devolutionary slide—at least in your own and your family's life.

After hearing all of this, you may be finding that it's difficult to remain hopeful about what is happening with our food supply, but I can tell you that more and more people are finding their way out of the maze. Change is in the air! So remember,

The actions you take may not appear to make much difference in the world.
But they have rippling effects—and influence the greater whole more
than you might ever imagine!

DIETARY DEVOLUTION #1

FROM FRUGIVORE TO OMNIVORE

We are a tropical species. We are also hominids, in the strictest sense of the word, which means *humans* and *relatives of humans* that are closer to us than chimpanzees. Humans are the only existing hominids, all others are extinct. Our anatomy still reflects that of other primates (apes & chimpanzees), who are our closest relatives in the animal world. For millions of years, hominids have eaten primarily fruit. Anthropologist Alan Walker of Johns Hopkins University confirmed this, through electron microscopy and other high-tech tools, from the examination of fossilized remains of early hominids.

Being natural fruit eaters, our earliest ancestors would have been guided by their sense of sight and smell to a sweet-tasting piece of fruit. They reached up to eat food from the trees, or plucked berries from shrubs and vines.

Sounds like paradise, doesn't it?

Scientists tell us that Homo sapiens have walked the earth less than 200,000 years, and during that time we have used tools to kill for meat. (This is especially true for those who wandered north or south to temperate and polar regions.) For this reason, there are those who view the human race as natural omnivores, rather than frugivores.

But it may be that archeologists have just scratched the surface of the multidimensional nature of our ancient history. There are myths and legends of great cities and high civilizations lost in the midst of time. There are records of astrophysical knowledge and technical feats, some of which we still cannot explain. The Hindu scriptures indicate that we had been on Earth four million years before The Great Deluge (the flood of Noah's time).

There are other sources of knowledge than the few fossil findings that have driven archeological speculations about the human past, and for diet in particular. For example, the ancient Greeks had interesting things to say about the diet of those who came before them, and that was not so long ago. Onomacritus of Athens (530-480 BC) said: "In the days before Lycurgus (the legendary lawmaker of Sparta, who is estimated to have lived around 800 BC), each generation reached the age of 200 years." A few centuries later, Plutarch (46-120 AD) observed: "The ancient Greeks, before the time of Lycurgus, ate nothing but fruits." We can deduce from these statements that the fruit-eaters were long-lived.

Various threads of a fruitarian diet are even woven throughout Greek historical accounts. The Pelasgians were the indigenous people who lived in the region of the Aegean Sea before the ancient Greek civilization arose. Hesiod (750-650 BC) said: "The Pelasgians and the peoples who came after them in Greece ate fruits of the virgin forests and blackberries from the fields."

A few centuries later, Philochorus (340-261 BC) said of the Pelasgians: "Their heroic spirit and their strong arms to destroy their foe were formed of shiny red apples from the forest. Apples were their favorite food, and the speed of their feet never lessened. They raced against stags and won. They lived for hundreds of years in the world of Cronus, but as they grew old, their vast stature never diminished, even by a thumb's breadth. The dark luster of their black hair was never tainted by a single silver thread."

In the first book of the Bible we read, "And God said, 'I have given you every plant with seeds on the face of the earth and every tree that has fruit with seeds. This will be your food.'" (Genesis 1:29.) In the days before The Flood, it was recorded that Methuselah, son of Enoch and the grandfather of Noah, lived to be 969 years of age. We cannot imagine it today, so we discount it, but what if we were meant to live much longer, healthier, and more productive lives? Regardless of whether you believe in the occurrence of these events, we can know one thing for sure: *we don't know what we don't know*. I know that sounds confusing, but think about it. We mostly relate to our world based on what we *think* we know about it. Our ideas and beliefs (repetitive thought forms) are the foundation of our experience, which is, then, limited by these very ideas and beliefs. So, I ask again: what if we were meant to live much longer, healthier, and more productive lives? What if we believed that *health* is our natural state, rather than disease?

Until very, very recently, most people lived according to their alkaline design, even among the hunter-gatherers who ate the meat of wild animals on occasion. Findings among fossil records of early hunter-gatherers and studies of contemporary people living a hunter-gatherer lifestyle show a high ratio of raw, alkalizing plant foods to animal flesh. This diet creates a state of "mild, systemic metabolic alkalosis"—alkaline values for blood, saliva, and urine. These findings by a group of clinical researchers from the University of California, among others, suggest that from an evolutionary perspective an alkaline condition is the natural and optimal state of health for humans.

But now a huge transformation has taken place in the human metabolic environment. Today, due to the devolution of our diet, human beings are mostly living in a mild to severe state of acidosis. In doing so, we are going against our natural, God-given design.

Many people have acquired a voracious appetite for meat. They have become cultural omnivores. They use tools to raise, kill, skin, drain the blood, disembowel and dismember, cook, season, process, and package the flesh of animals, before they eat it.

The modern omnivore diet consists of: cooked meats of domesticated animals; animal products such as eggs and milk products (not ever part of a hunter-gatherer lifestyle); cooked vegetables, grains, and beans; and an occasional salad or piece of fruit. In this scenario, meat, animal products, and grains are foremost, with a few side dishes of cooked, plant-derived mush. The modern omnivore diet not only tips but it crashes the scale from alkaline to acid. Here is a look at how the portions on the plate of a frugivore have been reversed by the modern cultural omnivore.

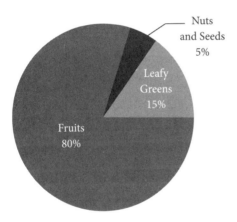

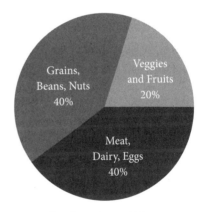

The Frugivore Diet　　　　　The Omnivore Diet

The move to an omnivorous diet, especially as practiced today, is a complete reversal of the frugivore diet. The majority of our original diet—the fruits of the trees—has been replaced by animal flesh and products, as well as grains, beans, nuts and legumes.

While humans may have adapted their diets to the conditions in which they found themselves throughout many millennia, my own experience of being a fruitarian throughout the majority of summer months (when fruit is plentiful) has shown me that a frugivore diet definitely brings about a clean, lean body, as well as a peaceful heart and clarity of mind.

After almost thirty-three years of experiencing every "healthy" diet possible—all raw for seven years, macrobiotic for two years, cooked vegetarian for five years, total frugivore during the summer months, I can honestly attest that a frugivore diet has had the most positive effect on both my consciousness and physical well-being.

WE ARE NOT DESIGNED TO EAT GRAINS

A big change took place with the Agricultural Revolution that began spreading around the world about 10,000 years ago. The domestication of animals and the cultivation of grains and legumes triggered the first great shift away from our alkaline design.

The fossil record indicates that the introduction of the agrarian diet coincided with a decline in human health. Prior to this time, there was no evidence of degenerative diseases or tooth decay. With the onset of settled communities and farms, however, people became shorter and sicker. There may have been all kinds of reasons for this—wars, lack of sanitation, the shake-up of societal structures—but diet likely played a huge part. Along with meat, milk, and eggs, people began to substitute seeds, including grains and beans, for fruits and greens.

The diet of those newly settled peoples was still much closer to nature than our contemporary diet. While we have access to a cornucopia of organic fruits and vegetables from our gardens and from the natural food store or farmer's markets, many people nevertheless eat few fresh fruits and vegetables.

The modern omnivore is a mix between a carnivore and a *grainivore*—an animal that feeds on the seeds of plants as a main food source. While animal products are difficult to digest, grains pose a variety of problems for our digestive system as well:

- They create mucus, similar to milk and dairy products.
- The most common grains—the glutinous ones—are extremely acid-forming.
- They do not have much nutrition for the amount of calories.
- They contain phytotoxins (another way of saying plant toxins), as do beans and other seeds.
- They contain high levels of phosphates (remember Lake Erie?)

Arnold Ehret, author of *The Mucusless Diet Healing System* (1922), was the first to speak of mucus as a primary carrier and substrate of diseases. As he described it, mucus is a kind of gluey, sticky substance that accumulates in the digestive tract over time when starchy foods, such as grains, are eaten. Dairy products (casein) and white flour (gluten) are the worst sources of mucus.

The glutinous grains have long been used in baking bread, the "staff of life." Unfortunately, bread as we know it is more likely to promote deterioration of the internal environment than strength and vitality.

According to Rhonda Nelson, ND, it is estimated that the hybridization and genetic engineering of wheat has resulted in a *500-fold* increase in the gluten content of today's wheat compared to the wheat our forefathers would have known. This may be one of the prime reasons behind the massive rise of gluten intolerance in recent decades.

Gluten intolerance is the name we give to a toxic, inflammatory buildup of mucoid plaque in the intestines, caused by mucus-forming foods and substances such as gluten in the diet. You'll remember that inflammation is a typical symptom of acidic, deoxygenated tissues. In case you want to know, mucoid plaque is "caked layers of hardened mucus mixed with fecal matter, bizarrely resembling hardened blackish-green truck tire rubber or an old piece of dried rawhide," as Richard Anderson, ND, founder of Arise and Shine Transformational Cleanse Programs, describes it.

At the core of fruits and vegetables are hundreds and thousands of powerful phytonutrients. Seeds, on the other hand, are dense bundles of caloric energy with some nutrients in the germ and bran, which are usually disposed of in making flours. The implications of this switch from plant flesh to plant seeds as the primary basis of our diet are huge.

Additionally, seeds have phytic acid in the outer or bran layer, as well as protease and enzyme inhibitors to prevent them from sprouting until conditions are right. They also block our body's assimilation of the nutrients in the seed.

You might be wondering whether grains can be a part of a healthy *EcoDiet*. I believe that a frugivore diet, which consists of fruits, tender greens and shoots, wild vegetation, and occasional nuts and seeds, can include a small amount of whole grains and beans while you are transitioning.

Here's how:

- Eat non-hybrid, heirloom grains and beans only.
- Change your diet with the seasons. Exclude grains completely during the warm months of the year. Only add a small amount of grains to your diet in the cold months.
- Never eat wheat. Focus on the non-glutinous, alkalizing pseudo-grains such as millet and quinoa, and the less common, heirloom grains and seeds such as chia, flax, and amaranth.
- Soak and rinse or sprout seeds before cooking or eating them raw. The seed "locks" that block the assimilation of nutrients are opened by water. Sprouting also vastly increases the protein content of the seed. It increases nutrients by 50 to 400%. What is actually happening, of course, is that you are transforming the seed into embryonic plant flesh!

Finally, while gluten intolerance has become a well-known syndrome, what about sensitivity to elevated phosphate levels? The omnivore staples of meat, dairy, eggs, grains, beans, and nuts are all phosphate-rich.

Dr. St. Amand tells us in his book *What Your Doctor May Not Tell You About Fibromyalgia* that fibromyalgia is a result of elevated levels of the wrong kinds of phosphate in the cells.

Hertha Hafer, a German research pharmacist, sees a link between elevated levels of phosphates, low pH, and neurological problems—ADD/ADHD syndromes in particular. Phosphorous is an important mineral and a natural, organic component of many foods. However, when phosphorous and phosphate compounds are consumed in large quantities, the calcium/phosphorous balance is disrupted, leading to deficiencies in mineral absorption. Of all the minerals, phosphate has the most influence on the body's pH regulatory system.

The solution? Lendon Smith, MD, an outspoken physician once known as "The Children's Doctor," wrote that the diet that best served the hyperactive child was "grazing, or nibbling, on raw fruits and vegetables."

BUT WHERE DO I GET MY PROTEIN?

One of the most common myths about a plant-based diet is that you will not get enough protein. The outdated myth that we have to consume meat for our daily requirements of protein has been completely invalidated.

Although protein is certainly an essential nutrient that plays many key roles in the way our bodies function, we do not need huge quantities of it as some schools teach. In fact, plant foods contain more than adequate amounts of protein.

As a comparison, one egg has 6 grams of protein. A medium avocado has 5 grams, a cup of cooked collard greens has 4 grams, a cup of cooked millet has 8.4 grams, and a cup of cooked lentils has 18 grams of protein. Not only does a plant-based diet provide adequate amounts of total dietary protein (about 10% total calories), these proteins are far superior to animal proteins.

Here's proof. In 2001, a group of endocrinologists at the University of California, San Francisco were wondering whether acidic, animal-protein sources would have different effects than alkaline, plant proteins. In fact, in a study of more than 1,000 elderly women, they found that a higher reliance on animal sources of protein significantly increased bone loss and the chances of hip fractures.

The China Study (2005) documents the results of the 20-year research project directed by medical researchers T. Colin Campbell, PhD, and Thomas M. Campbell II, in a partnership between Cornell University, Oxford University, and the Chinese Academy of Preventive Medicine. They compared the results of that study with a number of other provocative studies. The *New York Times* called it the "most comprehensive large study ever undertaken of the relationship between diet and the risk of developing disease."

The research project revealed that people who primarily ate animal-based foods developed more chronic diseases while people who primarily ate plant-based foods were healthier. They found abundant evidence linking diets high in protein, particularly animal protein (including casein in cow's milk), to chronic degenerative diseases. They go so far as to say "even relatively small intakes of animal-based foods were associated with adverse effects."

To test his theory about dairy products, Dr. Campbell fed two groups of rats diets with different amounts of casein, the main protein in dairy products. After 12 weeks, all of the rats eating a diet of 20% casein had a greatly increased level of early cancer tumor growth while rats eating a 5% diet showed no evidence of cancer. He discovered that cancer growth could be turned on and off just by adjusting the level of intake of milk protein.

A study of more than 500,000 middle-aged and elderly Americans led by Rashmi Sinha of the National Cancer Institute revealed that eating red meat increases the chances of dying prematurely. The equivalent of about a small hamburger every day was enough to significantly increase the risk of premature death—mostly from heart disease and cancer—during the ten years that the study participants were followed. Sausage, cold cuts, and other processed meats also increased the risk.

Pork is perhaps the most problematic of common animal meats because the pig is biologically similar to humans. This means that many pathogens can be passed between pigs and people, and contracted from the consumption of pork. According to Paul Jaminet, co-author of *Perfect Health Diet*, one of those pathogens is the hepatitis E virus, which may be responsible for the three most common diseases associated with pork consumption—liver cirrhosis, liver cancer, and multiple sclerosis. So, if you choose to eat meat, consider at least staying away from pork.

Want to save our planet?

STOP EATING MEAT!

Another major factor to consider in the devolutionary shift from a frugivore diet to our modern omnivore diet is the devastation of our planet.

A 2006 United Nations report summarized the devastation caused by the meat industry by calling it "one of the top two or three most significant contributors to the most serious environmental problems, at every scale from local to global." The report recommended animal agriculture as "a major policy focus when dealing with problems of land degradation, climate change and air pollution, water shortage and water pollution, and loss of biodiversity."

The livestock industry takes up 70% of agricultural land and is largely responsible for deforestation. Over half of the greenhouse gases responsible for global warming come from livestock operations…and that's just the beginning.

One of the greatest things you can do in your everyday life to save the environment is to eat an alkaline, plant-based diet. It makes a greater difference than driving a fuel-efficient car, for instance. A University of Chicago study determined that in terms of fossil-fuel consumption, there is a large order-of-magnitude difference between dietary choices and what you drive. In other words, your daily food choices have a much greater impact.

A global solution for both our inner and outer environmental crises could be as simple as this: eliminate the consumption of animals and animal products and become the frugivores we were created to be.

DIETARY DEVOLUTION #2
FROM OMNIVORE TO CHEMIVORE

Carnivores feed from the top of the food chain. Omnivores also feed in part from the top of the food chain. Since the industrial revolution, eating from the top of the food chain has taken an even more disturbing turn. Let's take a look at how chemicals have permeated every part of our planet's environment as well as the environment of the human body, and how eating foods from the top of the food chain are hazardous to your health!

HOW CHEMICALS ENTER THE FOOD CHAIN

In recent years, arctic waters, while once relatively pristine, are becoming toxic. Chemicals from the fall-out of agriculture, jet exhaust, and industrial manufacturing plants, along with the burning of fossil fuel, have reached the farthest corners of the earth, carried by rivers, ocean currents, and winds.

Aquatic life in the Arctic feed from plankton, and plankton derives its nutrients from the waters of the ocean. In the process of collecting nutrients (a process called *bioaccumulation*), toxic pollutants are also accumulated, making the pollutants much more concentrated in the cells of the plankton than in the open water.

Because small fish eat vast amounts of plankton, these toxic chemicals collect and concentrate in their flesh. This process is called *biomagnification* and is repeated at each step of the food chain. Predators four to five links up on the food chain are found to have accumulations of toxic chemicals in their tissues millions of times higher than that of the water they inhabit. The same principles apply to land animals, of course.

Greenlanders traditionally eat almost entirely from the sea, and I do not mean seaweed. They eat from the top of the food chain, fish and other marine life. Tragically, scientists are finding hundreds of hazardous synthetic compounds in the flesh of people who inhabit the Arctic tundra, at levels so extreme that the breast milk and tissues of some Greenlander people could be classified as hazardous waste.

The same principles of bioaccumulation and biomagnification apply to land animals, of course. The meat of farm animals, as well as wild life, contains concentrated levels of toxins from contaminated feed and the toxic fields in which they graze. These days, to eat meat is to take your life in your hands.

Want to lose weight?
STOP EATING TOXIC MEAT

Toxic chemicals can make you fat. Toxins interfere with our metabolic systems and cause us to store fat. This may be in part because the body uses fat cells for storing toxins it cannot easily eliminate. The body then resists breaking down fat cells in an attempt to protect itself from autointoxication, as described in the previous section.

Paula Baille-Hamilton, MD reports that toxic chemicals such as organophosphates, carbamates, anti-thyroid drugs, steroids, antibiotics, and organochlorines are fed to our livestock. Such toxic classes of chemicals interfere with the weight-regulating hormones in cattle—and in humans. They are added to cattle feed in minute amounts—not enough to make the animals really ill, just fat!

Through bioaccumulation (from feed) and biomagnification (in the case of animals fed on the carcasses of other animals, which include feces, as well as toxic chemicals), these toxins are highly concentrated and end up on our plates as part of the steak or hamburger.

Bottom line: Toxic chemicals make you fat! So, if you want to lose weight, get off the chemical fatteners! If you must eat meat, eat the meat of organic, pasture-raised animals. Better yet, eat an organic, plant-based diet!

Want to avoid cancer?
CUT OUT THE COLD CUTS

Deli meats, lunchmeats, cold cuts, bologna—whatever you call it, are processed meats. Hot dogs, spam and bacon also belong in this category. In addition to the environmental toxins and the chemicals that are intentionally fed to animals, there are the chemical additives that are mixed into processed meats. One of the additives commonly used in these processed meats is nitrates or nitrites. Nitrites are used to artificially preserve the pink color of the meat so it won't turn grey, and to help prevent botulism.

During the processing of these meats, nitrites combine with amines (organic compounds of nitrogen) in the meat to form carcinogenic compounds. Not unexpectedly, studies of people who eat processed meats have shown a greater likelihood of contracting cancer.

Still want to eat meat?
AVOID FACTORY-RAISED MEAT

The way in which we care for animals also has an effect on our own health and well-being. The industrialization of animal husbandry, in which animals are treated merely as units of production, affects us in deep ways. When a living being is subjected to high levels of physical, chemical, emotional and mental stress, and suffering, the body reflects that. There are chemical stress signals: hormones are affected, metabolism is altered, and disease mechanisms are triggered. When we eat the flesh of these animals, we are eating the architecture of their suffering.

Moreover, when we support the egregious practice of factory farming by purchasing meat from markets, we are participating in the on-going suffering of animals, and on a deep level this affects us. Remember, as I said earlier, our true nature is to be loving and cooperative; we are one with all of life whether we realize it or not. In the words of anti-apartheid activist, revolutionary and politician Nelson Mandela: "For to be free is not merely to cast off one's chains, but to live in a way that respects and enhances the freedom of others."

STOP EATING FROM TOXIC OCEANS

Radiation

Since the nuclear reactor meltdowns in Fukushima, Japan, radioactive contamination of seafood is becoming a real issue.

Pacific Bluefin tuna spawn off the coast of Japan and swim across the ocean to school in the waters along the coast of California and the tip of Baja California, Mexico. In May 2012, a report in the *Huffington Post* revealed that levels of radioactive cesium in these great fish were 10 times higher than usual.

Sea vegetables (aka seaweeds), like the fish of the sea, have also come under suspicion of radioactive contamination. Since the Fukushima nuclear power plant meltdowns in Japan, there have been reports of radiation-contaminated sea vegetables being sold in the United States. Michael Collins, writing for *EnviroReporter* on April 20, 2012, reports:

> On April 13, 2012 *EnviroReporter.com* tested *Nori* seaweed from Japan bought in a West Los Angeles store, the same one where this reporter bought the identical item eight months ago soon after the Fukushima Daiichi meltdowns began in Japan. The trendy and 'organic' delicacy, popular with LA hipsters, was 94.7% above normal, 17.6% of that additional ionization indicative of alpha radiation which can be 60 to 1,000 times more dangerous than beta and gamma radiation.

He also notes that it is possible for the Japanese to export radiation-contaminated food products that do not meet their standards to the United States, which has "standards up to dozens of times more lax" for the kinds of radioactive particles spewing out of the nuclear plants in Fukushima.

It has become important to check on the source of sea vegetables. Not all sea vegetables from Japan are contaminated, but some may be. For now, I would recommend buying from highly reputable sources like Maine Coast Sea Vegetables. Uncontaminated sea vegetables are a great source of iodine and are great for detoxifying radioactive substances from the body.

Mercury

Yet another factor to consider in eating fish is mercury toxicity. Have you ever wondered how mercury ends up in fish? Look to the coal industry, as coal contains some mercury. When coal is burned in power plants for electricity, that mercury goes out the stack. It eventually falls to the earth, or the ocean, in our rain. It is taken up along with nutrients from the sea in the growth of plankton. Small fish feed on the plankton and are eaten by larger fish, which are eaten by yet larger fish, which are then eaten by people. What goes around comes around, as they say. Here is a simple illustration of how it works.

How mercury makes its way into the environment

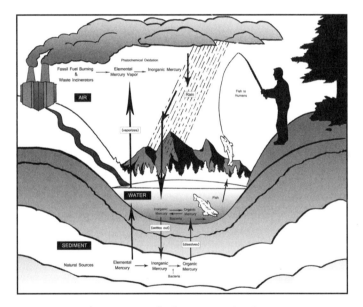

Source: *http://www.mercury.utah.gov/atmospheric_transport.html*

Some people believe that eating farm-raised fish is a healthy choice, and there's no reason it couldn't be. But, unfortunately, in our industrialized world, farm-raised fish are much more contaminated than the already extremely contaminated wild fish.

Studies in 2004 and 2005 showed farm-raised salmon with higher levels of mercury and 10 or 11 times higher levels of carcinogens than wild-caught fish. To complicate matters, much of the fish that is labeled "wild-caught" is actually farm-raise, due to loopholes in the law and lax enforcement by the USDA.

But if you still want to include fish in your diet, you may want to consider fish that are lower on the food chain and wild-caught: mackerel, sardines, herring, oysters, and shrimp, for instance. Remove the skin. Realize though that when you fish and eat species in which mercury and other toxins are less concentrated, we are also removing the food sources of larger, longer-lived fish like tuna, cod, and snapper, thereby causing breakdowns in marine ecosystems. It is a no-win situation. Ending pollution, cleaning up the oceans, and switching to a plant-based diet is the only real answer.

STOP CONSUMING DAIRY PRODUCTS

First, there are the chemical contaminants like drugs, pesticide-laced feed, and growth hormones that enter the milk from industrial farming practices. In addition, pasteurization and homogenization both profoundly alter the chemical structure of milk, making it a food unfit for human consumption.

The common practice of pasteurization involves heating milk to 145 °F for 30 minutes or 163 °F for 15 seconds (called *flash pasteurization*). The use of heat to destroy objectionable bacteria also destroys enzymes, beneficial bacteria, and nutrients.

Homogenization is a process whereby milk is pushed through a fine filter at pressures of 4,000 pounds per square inch. The structure of the milk proteins is changed—degraded, actually.

Homogenization is used to create uniformity of flavor and fat content in large batches of milk. It keeps the cream from separating and rising to the top.

The health dangers of pasteurized and homogenized milk are:

- Processing the milk kills beneficial bacteria, leaving large batches of milk susceptible to environmental contamination by pathogenic bacteria, and large outbreaks of illness are more common than we realize.
- Processing the milk destroys enzymes and vitamins—especially C, B6 and B12, and alters milk proteins, making them less digestible.
- Calcium in the milk is less available, due to altered milk fats and destruction of enzymes.

- May contain assorted drugs and antibiotics, pesticides from treated grains, bacteria from infected animals, and genetically engineered growth hormones (rBST or BGH).
- Associated with diminished resistance to disease, increased risk of bone fractures, and high cholesterol.
- Known for its role in triggering health problems such as allergies, nasal congestion, constipation, increased tooth decay, anemia, arthritis, osteoporosis, atherosclerosis, leukemia, prostate cancer, ovarian cancer, nephrosis, heart disease.
- Can trigger autoimmune diseases such as diabetes, Lou Gehrig's disease, or Multiple Sclerosis.
- Associated with infant and childhood illnesses such as ear infections, strep infections, colic, iron-deficiency anemia, asthma, growth problems, and anti-social behavior.

Most people believe that milk stamped with an organic certification assures a higher standard. Unfortunately, this is not always true. Organic milk in the grocery stores is mostly ultra-pasteurized. Ultra-pasteurization does even more damage to milk than the usual process of pasteurization. The plastic or plastic-lined packaging also leaches various endocrine-disrupting compounds into the milk. Thus, organic, ultra-pasteurized milk falls squarely into the *chemivore* level of dietary devolution.

Milk found on grocery-store shelves today is very different from what our farming ancestors drank. Raw milk that comes from cows that graze on green pastures is a slightly alkaline food. This is because cows eat grass, which is highly alkaline. But it is high in fat, so why not get your chlorophyll first hand from low-fat sources such as fruits and leafy greens?

Did you know that milk comes in two varieties? They are known as A1 and A2. A1 and A2 refer to a minor difference in the position of an amino acid in beta casein, the protein in milk. Until about five thousand years ago, there was only one type of milk, what we call A2. Then, a genetic mutation occurred in some cattle, and they began to produce A1 milk. Some cows today still produce A2 milk, but most of the dairy cows in the United States are producers of A1 milk. Though the genetic difference is very slight, the effects are significant.

A New Zealand study called the Fonterra Study found that neurological and mental disorders could be induced or aggravated by drinking A1 milk. There's also some evidence showing associations between the A1 casein in milk and increased risk of heart disease and diabetes. Drinking A2 milk did not have the same disease-causing effects.

If you want to drink milk, consider raw goat milk. All goat milk is A2. If you use the high-fat milk products such as cream or butter, purchase goat milk products, if possible, and be sure to go organic. Even though it can be more expensive, it is worth it for the sake of your health. Chemical toxins, including pesticides, are bioaccumulated and biomagnified in dairy products too, especially the fatty portion of the milk—the cream and the butter made from that cream.

This is because most modern industrial chemicals, including pesticides and drugs, are derived from petroleum (oil)! In pumping oil from underground veins, one could say that we are extracting the "fat of the land." Chemicals that are created from this fat of the land are *fat-soluble* (requiring fats for digestion and absorption rather than water) and, therefore, end up in the fatty portions of animal products and in our fatty tissues.

STOP EATING FOOD FROM TOXIC FIELDS

Our agriculture and food supply is now characterized by:

- intensive, widespread irrigation on marginal, depleted soils;
- chemically intensive cropping;
- genetic engineering of seed;
- centralization of ownership and distribution in a few hands;
- long shipping distances;
- chemical additives, preservatives, and irradiation; and,
- poor flavor and lower levels of nutrients.

Agriculture as we know it today is not sustainable. It is consumer agriculture—consuming resources without replenishing them. As with the extraction of oil in the fossil fuel industry, resources of land and water are being used up at an incredible rate.

Billions of pounds of chemicals are applied to the land in an attempt to prop up soil fertility and reduce destruction to crops from pests. The result is the destruction of the microbial life of the soil and beneficial insects, including bees and butterflies.

Toxic pesticides that have been banned for use here are still used on crops in various foreign countries. For example, many fruits and vegetables are imported from Mexico, especially in the wintertime. Sadly, only a small percentage of the billions of pounds of food imported into the United States are inspected for pesticide residues.

Pesticide and fungicide residues and waxes are very difficult to wash off of fruits and vegetables, and peeling off the skin does not keep us safe either, as chemical residues are often absorbed into the flesh of the produce. Then, there are insecticides that are part of the plant's genetic structure, like Bt-toxins in Monsanto's (one of America's leading multinational chemical conglomerates) genetically modified sweet corn. Can't wash those off!

There is a growing body of research on petroleum-based chemicals and pesticides. Pesticides have been shown to cause significant weakening effects to the nervous system and immune system. Illnesses identified in the medical research include adult and child cancers, numerous neurological disorders, immune system weakening, autoimmune disorders, asthma, allergies, infertility, miscarriage, and child behavior disorders, including learning disabilities, mental retardation, hyperactivity, and attention deficit disorders (ADD). These are just some of the effects of toxic load and chronic acidosis.

Identifying a specific chemical (or mycotoxin, *see below*) as the original cause of health disorders in the general population is difficult and often overlooked, as it typically requires years of exposure for the body's inherent defenses to weaken sufficiently to result in observable health problems. Also, many of our illnesses are a result of a combination of petroleum-based, chemicals working in tandem, making specific identification even more difficult.

Paula Baillie-Hamilton, MD, author of *The Body Restoration Plan*, notes that the ever-increasing role of petroleum as a basis of our society through the last century parallels the ever-increasing role of acidosis as a basis of the diseases from which we suffer.

The Growing Problem of Mycotoxins

Like the invasive forms of candida, other forms of fungi can also exude poisonous substances, called mycotoxins. Toxic fields spawn mycotoxins.

Higher levels of mycotoxins have been reported in grains grown under high-yield, chemical-intensive farming systems. In a study by The Organic Center on matched pairs of foods, mycotoxins were a more serious issue in the conventionally grown foods—twice as often at levels twice as high.

Are conventionally farmed fields moldier?

Synthetic nitrogen fertilizer stimulates higher levels of fungal growth. When fertilizer-stimulated fungal populations come under stress from bad weather or other environmental difficulties, they produce mycotoxins as a part of their survival response.

Then, there's the really big problem. Monsanto's favorite organophosphate herbicide, and the most widely used herbicide in the world, Round-up® (common name glyphosate) can accumulate and persist in the soil for years. Our extensive use of Round-up in the last thirty years has destroyed the balance of microbes in our agricultural soils, and locked up soil nutrients, meaning that they are no longer available to plants. Microbes are to the soil what friendly bacteria are to your intestinal tract.

Round-up not only destroys protective bacteria in soil, it also promotes more aggressive and virulent pathogens—the family of fungi known as *Fusarium*, in particular. Applications of fungicide to control the eruptions of fungi from applications of Round-up can trigger further mycotoxin outbreaks in field crops. This is because applying fungicide doesn't instantly kill all of the fungus in a field. The fungus that doesn't die immediately is highly stressed, and its defense mechanisms move into high gear with an explosion of mycotoxins.

What we have with glyphosate is the most abused chemical
we have ever had in the history of man.

—Dr. Don Huber, Professor Emeritus of Plant Pathology at Purdue University

When applied to crops, Round-up becomes systemic throughout the plant, so it cannot be washed off. And once you eat this plant, or its seed, the glyphosate ends up in your gut where it can decimate your beneficial bacteria, just as it does the beneficial microbes in the soil. This is the case for all crops grown with Round-up, not just "Round-Up Ready" GMOs.

The genus Fusarium creates more than a dozen known mycotoxins, which especially affect the nervous and endocrine systems. In talking about Round-up, plant pathologist Don Huber says, "You look at Alzheimer's, thyroid problems, autism, Parkinson's—any of those diseases that have a tie with either the endocrine system or nutrient availability. We're going to see those [diseases] increase."

Round-up and glyphosate marketed by various other names—produces a double whammy: (1) the direct effect of the chemical residue in our intestinal tract, which destroys the balance of microorganisms and reduces nutrient bioavailability, and (2) the Round-up-stimulated fungal mycotoxins and their various, deadly, systemic effects.

In 2007, the USDA asked for permission to stop recording how much glyphosate we use. Don Huber remarks, "It was going up so rapidly that it was embarrassing, I think, for anybody to realize how much of this organic phosphate was being put out ....We're seeing the effect on organisms in the intestinal tract just from the residue in the food and feeds."

You could say, perhaps, that mycotoxins are the "stress hormones" of the soil kingdom. Exceedingly low concentrations of mycotoxins (parts per billion) can have devastating effects when ingested. They are particularly known for disrupting the endocrine system. This has certain logic since our endocrine system is involved in the management of stress and trauma. By eating the chemical stress signals of the soil, we take it upon ourselves. We can expect that mycotoxins will have various effects in the body similar to our own chemical stress signals.

Needless to say, mycotoxins are not only a problem in the field, but can also arise from mold growth in the storage of grains and other foods. Fungal infestations and their poisonous excretions are also a growing problem in our homes and businesses.

Pathological fungus and molds can gain a greater foothold in deoxygenated areas. For a mold-free body, keep your friendly intestinal populations strong and happy in an alkaline and oxygen-rich environment, fed by fresh, organic fruits and vegetables!

WANT PRODUCE WITH LOTS OF NUTRIENTS?
Eat Organic

Organic is a term used for foods that have been grown without the use of synthetic fertilizers and pesticides, and with non-GMO seeds. If possible, buy foods that are certified by independent organizations like QAI, Oregon Tilth, and CCOF. USDA Organic standards are much lower.

Biodynamic is a term used for foods organically grown according to the spiritual science revealed by Rudolf Steiner (1861-1925). Biodynamic farming goes further in its approach to sustainable farming. It uses what some would call unorthodox methodologies to create the most nutritious foods possible. Biodynamic farmers apply homeopathic field sprays and herbal compost preparations at certain seasons and phases of the moon, for example.

One of the biggest complaints that people have in purchasing organic or biodynamic produce is that it generally costs more than conventional produce. If you are on a budget it can be discouraging. However, consider this: a new study shows the superior nutritional value of organically grown produce.

According to a recent four-year $25 million European Union–funded study, organic food is, in fact, more nutritious than conventional produce and may be better at preventing cancer and heart disease. Researchers found that fruits and vegetables contain up to 40% more antioxidants if they are grown without chemical fertilizers and pesticides.

Just keep this in mind when you're at the check-out line: you may be paying a little more for that biodynamic or organically grown tomato, but it may take two conventionally grown tomatoes to match up with the nutritional value of one organically grown tomato.

Think nutrient density! Minimize chemical and mycotoxic load! Consider eating less food, but food of higher quality!

Cannot find organic produce?
BUY LOW ON THE PESTICIDE FOOD CHAIN

If you live in an area where it is difficult to find organic fruits and vegetables, you may need to limit your exposure to pesticides by buying low on the pesticide chain. The Environmental Working Group lists foods by pesticide exposure from highest to lowest. In 2012, the highest risks of multiple pesticide exposures were shown in the following foods.

They call them the "dirty dozen":

Apples	Celery	Grapes	Bell Peppers
Strawberries	Peaches	Potatoes	Blueberries
Spinach	Nectarines	Lettuce	Kale and Collards

The cleanest conventionally grown foods—that is, the lowest on the pesticide chain, were:

Onions	Avocado	Asparagus	Sweet peas
Mangoes	Eggplant	Cantaloupe	Kiwi
Cabbage	Watermelon	Sweet potatoes	Grapefruit

If you can't buy organic at your local grocery store, try eliminating the dirty dozen from your diet. Remember, because of bioaccumulation and biomagnification, the most important foods to buy organic, if you eat them, are animal flesh, eggs, and dairy products.

Other options include:

- Grow your own with heirloom seeds.
- Shop at your local farmer's market and natural food co-op.
- Join a CSA or make a deal with a local, sustainable farmer or gardener.
- Join a local cooperative food-buying club for organic products.
- Join an online membership organization like Green Polka Dot Box to have organic foods (even fresh produce!) shipped directly to your door at discounted prices!

STOP EATING IRRADIATED FOODS

One of the latest additions to chemical devolution is the exposure of our food to radioactivity to extend its shipping or shelf life. Foods being irradiated include meats, grains, herbs, and produce.

Irradiated food is generally bombarded with radiation 5 thousand to 1 million times greater than a chest x-ray.

The results of this exposure in foods include:

- creation of free radicals;
- damage to nutrients (may lose up to 80% of vitamins);
- damage to enzymes;
- creation of unique radiolytic (chemical breakdown due to radiation) products (some of these chemical by-products are known toxins and some are unique to irradiated foods, their effects as yet undocumented);
- tendency of fat to become rancid;
- damage to the DNA of the living cells of the food;
- trace amounts of lingering radioactivity.

Raw foods that have been irradiated look just like fresh foods, but nutritionally they are more like cooked foods, with decreased vitamins and enzymes. Still, the FDA allows these foods to be labeled fresh.

Treating solid foods with radiation provides an effect similar to heat pasteurization of liquids, such as milk. While irradiation is a fundamentally different process, ironically, there are those who use the term cold pasteurization to describe the irradiation of foods.

It is hard to say how widespread irradiation is, but many restaurants and pretty much all fast-food outlets use irradiated foods. Many items in the grocery store include irradiated ingredients. If an entire product is irradiated, the symbol for irradiation, the radura, should be shown on the product's package. However, when irradiated food is used as an ingredient in a product, the symbol is not required.

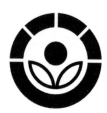

STOP THE GMO DEVOLUTION MADNESS

Genetic engineering involves taking genes from one strain of a plant, animal, or microorganism and inserting them into another with the goal of introducing desired characteristics, such as increasing a plant's resistance to insects, or enhancing the sweetness of a fruit. The practice is undertaken in part for economic reasons; if genetically modified plants become more resistant to harmful microbes and insects, yields are improved.

However, bits of genetic materials from organisms that have never been a part of the human food supply are changing the fundamental nature of the food we eat. Thus, when a plant's genes are manipulated, the result is no longer a plant, due to animal, fungus, and mutated genes mixed into it. It is a *genetically modified organism* (GMO).

Arpad Pusztai, one of the first scientists to raise concerns about the safety of genetically modified foods, has this to say:

> Gene insertion is a major problem. You cannot direct where the splicing of the genetic construct will happen. It is well known that when you insert a genetic construct into the DNA network of a plant, you create changes in that network. As a result, you will get changes in the functionality of the plant's own genes. They may become more active or silent. The effects will be unpredictable and uncontrollable. It can sometimes cause irreparable damage to the genome. This is called *insertional mutagenesis.*

In other words, the practice of genetic modification creates unpredictable, uncontrollable, and sometimes irreparable damage to the genome. Biotech scientists are experimenting with very delicate, yet powerful forces of nature without full knowledge of the widespread repercussions. Without long-term testing, no one knows if these foods are safe.

Here's an example that illustrates the politics of GMOs: Research published in the *International Journal of Biological Sciences* (2009) showed that three varieties of genetically modified corn caused organ damage in rats. (There were no human studies.) All three varieties had been approved by numerous food safety authorities and are widely available in the United States, Europe, and elsewhere.

These were all Monsanto varieties. As mentioned earlier, Monsanto is one of the largest (multiple-billion dollar) biotechnology corporations in the world developing and patenting genetically engineered seeds. The data used by Monsanto for the approval of these GMO varieties, ironically, is the same raw data that independent researchers studied to make the organ-damage link. They found serious mistakes in Monsanto's analysis of the data.

And, in case you are wondering, these GMO varieties are still on the market, along with several new varieties of GMO corn, including sweet corn.

Unraveling the Genetic Strand

Pesticides and other toxins generally diminish over time when left in the environment. Even if it takes a long time, eventually, they will break down into less harmful compounds. Unlike most toxins, when GMOs are released into the environment, they do not revert to their original nature over time. Instead, they have the effect of unraveling and corrupting the genetic integrity of all life, especially those families of life to which they are closely related.

Experience has shown that a small release from a field of GMO canola plants, for instance, will increase its presence in nearby non-GMO canola fields each following season. The GMO canola will also cross-pollinate with nearby weeds of similar botanical families. When these weeds re-grow from seed the next season, they are now also genetically modified. Even small amounts of GMO contamination will take over large areas and families of plants over time, with no end in sight.

Irradiation and genetic modification have in common the introduction of "strange chemistry," both known and unknown, through changes in the deep molecular structure of the seed, plant, fruit, meat, eggs or milk. They wreak havoc by changing the original nature of our food from within.

GMO, in my opinion, stands for *Godlessly Modified Organisms*, since we are changing the genetic signature of a species as originally created by God. The blueprint of these species is not being changed by natural evolution, or even by selective breeding, but by bombardment of the DNA by a group of people who are playing God. When man thinks that it knows better than the Creator and the creation itself, it means trouble. We have no idea what this adulteration will lead to.

Ultimately, in our callous willingness to manipulate other forms of life, we may be putting our own "seed"—the seeds of future generations—at risk.

Want to avoid GMOs?

EAT ORGANIC

I wish I could say to *eat organic* with absolute confidence. Unfortunately, the organic industry is under siege by GMO contamination in the fields, lack of enforcement by USDA, and intense regulatory lobbying by large, industrial growers.

Large corporations like Pepsi and Kraft Foods, who are far removed from the basic principles of integrity that underlie the organic movement, own many organic brands. Pepsi, the owner of organic and natural brands such as Naked Juice and Tazo teas, gave over $2 million to defeat the 2012 GMO labeling initiative in California, which would have made it mandatory for corporations to identify GMO-ingredients on food labels. Without the regulation, consumers cannot know for sure if the products they are consuming are non-GMO products.

In March 2012, the National Organic Standards Board wrote a letter to the USDA about their concerns. Included in that letter was the statement, "The NOSB, speaking for the organic community, believes the USDA's actions on genetically engineered crops have been insufficient to protect the organic industry."

Still, for now, organic is the best assurance we have. Be sure to buy *100% certified organic*. An *organic* label (certified organic, USDA organic) that does not say *100% organic* may still include—by law— 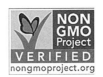 5% non-organic or GMO ingredients. *Made with Organic* labels need only contain 70% organic ingredients, so 30% could be GMO. You can also look for a Non-GMO Project Verified seal.

Another way to avoid GMO foods is to simply avoid known GMO crops. The big five are soy, corn, canola, cottonseed, and beet sugar. Unless it is specifically listed as cane sugar, sugar is likely to be GMO beet sugar. To stay up to date with GMOs, go to NonGMOShoppingGuide.com and download the shopping guide.

DIETARY DEVOLUTION #3

FROM CHEMIVORE TO JUNKIVORE

According to the USDA's Economic Research Service (ERS) food expenditure statistics, Americans spend about 10% of their disposable income on food. Regrettably, 90% of those dollars are spent on high-calorie, nutrient-deprived, processed junk foods loaded with toxic chemicals. This means that most Americans have become *junkivores!*

Buyer beware: Did you know?

- The commercial food industry adds over 1,000 new chemicals into our food supply each and every year.
- The average American consumes more than five pounds of chemicals each year from the food they eat.
- The FDA allows the term "natural" on food labels, provided the product is free of artificial flavors, chemical preservatives, or added colors.
- GMOs and irradiated foods may be legally labeled as natural!

Our food supply has devolved even further with the production of empty-calorie junk foods. Junk foods are junk—some of the most environmentally unfriendly, acidifying foods of all.

There are food companies that create products with the cheapest food-like substances possible—fake foods that seduce us with bright, chemical colors, corrupt our taste buds, and boast a long shelf life. These fake foods appeal more to our wounded psyches and addictions than to the true need and desire for nourishment.

Junk foods are characterized by:

- highly processed starches, like potatoes and grains.
- highly processed salt, oil, and sugar.
- artificial colors and flavors.
- artificial sweeteners.
- chemical preservatives.
- GMO-derived chemical additives.
- petroleum-based, chemical replacements for food ingredients.
- numerous other man-made, petroleum-based ingredients to help in the manufacturing, appearance, texture, and shelf life of the product.

My Motto:
If you can't read it, don't eat it!

Take a look at a list of the toxic chemicals included in the strawberry flavoring of a milkshake served at a fast-food drive-thru window:

> Amyl acetate, amyl butyrate, amyl valerate, anethol, anisyl formate, benzyl acetate, benzyl isobutyrate, butyric acid, cinnamyl isobutyrate, cinnamylvalerate, cognac essential oil, diacetyl, dipropyl ketone, ethyl butyrate, ethyl cinnamate, ethyl heptanoate, ethyl lactate, ethyl methylphenylglycidate, ethyl nitrate, ethyl propionate, ethyl valerbate, heliotropin, hydroxphrenyl-2butanone (10% solution to alcohol), a-ionone, isobutyl anthranilate, isobutyl butrate, lemon essential oil, maltol, 4-methylacetophenone, methyl anthranilate, methyl benzoate, methyl cinnamate, methyl heptine carbone, methyl naphthyl ketone, methyl slicylate, mint essential oil, neroli essential oil, nerolin, neryl isobulyrate, orris butter, phenethyl alcohol, sore rum ether, g-undecalctone, vanillin, and solvent 3.

Talk about fake food! I marvel at what it must have taken to create a formula of mostly synthetic chemicals to mimic the flavor and texture of actual food. What would be the motivation? Perhaps, if it can be created in a manufacturing setting from the raw material of petroleum, then there's no need to submit to the vagaries of the weather and the unpredictability of living beings. Something is lost, though, don't you think?

STOP EATING EMPTY CALORIES

The junkivore diet is problematic not only for what it contains, but also for what it does not contain. These are foods that promise but don't deliver.

In nature, a sweet flavor is usually a sign of ripeness, which means that the nutrients of the fruit or vegetable are at their optimum value. In soda pop, there's the promise of sweetness, but no nutrient delivery.

Many who have slipped into the junkivore diet are malnourished because of this lack of delivery. Junkivores tend to be hungry a lot, snacking through the day because they can't wait for the next meal. They may be metabolically compromised, with blood-sugar highs and lows, or diabetes. Many junk-food eaters are overweight. Constantly hungering for something to satisfy, they feed the addictive craving, but end up with very little in the way of actual nourishment.

Mark Hyman, MD, speaks and writes about the shocking fact that Americans are suffering from massive nutritional deficiencies.

> What I see in my office is reflected in the scientific literature. Upwards of 30% of American diets fall short of such common plant-derived nutrients as magnesium, vitamin C, vitamin E, and vitamin A. More than 80% of Americans are running low on vitamin D, and nine out of 10 people are deficient in omega-3 fats, which are critical for staving off inflammation and controlling blood sugar levels.

In less than a decade, America has gone from one in ten kids to almost one in four kids with pre-diabetes or diabetes. However, while obesity is often a sign of malnutrition, you can be slim and trim, looking good, and still be malnourished. For example, in a recent study of teenagers between the ages of 12 and 19, 23% were either pre-diabetic or diabetic. Most of these kids fit the general profile of being overweight, but 13% of the children in this at-risk group were of normal weight.

What Foods Are You Craving?

- A fresh-pressed apple-ginger-lemon juice, a raw soup (avocado pit included), a kale salad with nasturtium flowers and an oil-free dressing (all organically grown, of course)?

- Fried chicken, mashed potatoes with chicken-fat gravy, and steamed asparagus?

- A glass of (pasteurized) milk, a salami sandwich, and a packaged iceberg lettuce salad with ranch dressing?

- A coke, a bag of chips, a cheeseburger?

- Your next dose of meds?

What you crave can tell you a lot about how profoundly your taste buds have been corrupted and the level of dietary devolution you are experiencing.

Perhaps you're thinking that a kale salad is just not the sort of thing a person craves. You might nibble at it because it is supposed to be good for you, but, really don't desire it.

If you are ready to change to a more organic, holistic, pure, nutrient-dense *EcoDiet,* it will take a little discipline, and a little time. It takes time to shift out of those old familiar, nutrient-void food habits. Then before you know it, your cells will "wake up" and say "thank you" for the newfound energy that is available to them. This is when *EcoDiet* becomes a lifestyle.

The biggest issue for most people is simply this: We use meat, fats, starches, and processed junk foods, and eventually drugs, to numb hurts and emotional pain. So, changing your diet is only one part of the equation, but it's a necessary and important part. If you really want to make a quantum shift, however, you will need to also address your internal environment by facing old emotional patterns and habitual and painful ways of being in life. The habits related to emotional pain are a significant part of the entrenchment of an acid internal environment. Without the resolve to heal the sources of your emotional pain, you may only be able to sustain a temporary shift in diet before slipping back into old ways.

As you are making the shift and beginning to live the *EcoDiet* lifestyle, you may have some experiences you didn't expect:

- The living glow of greens and fruits at the farmer's market dazzles you and creates within you a profound joy.
- You dream about the next fresh juice you're going to make—with great satisfaction.
- The thought of a salad becomes satisfying.
- You eat less—naturally.
- You don't feel as hungry. In fact, you may even skip a meal now and then without noticing any hunger or faintness.
- You feel a deep sense of gratitude for the living fruits and vegetables that have become your food.
- You fall off the wagon and eat a sugar cookie. But interestingly, while the first two or three bites are quite tasty, after that, it fails to satisfy.

- You take a bite of meat. The texture between your teeth and the realization that you are eating flesh is slightly nauseating.

These are all signs that you are regaining a sense of what it means to be eating the foods you were designed to eat—foods that truly nourish you.

FAKE FOODS

Our sense of taste is intended to guide us in our food choices so that we can choose the most nourishing foods. In a world that supports our greatest health, the things that taste best on the tongue and trigger our salivary glands to secrete digestive juices would also be the healthiest. However, we have managed to subvert the natural, normal sense of taste, and to trick it into desiring many things that are bad for us. Time after time, we "bite" on the promises that don't deliver. We crave foods that don't ultimately satisfy. We also end up living lives that reflect this sad trend.

MSG, Aspartame, and Olestra are powerful chemicals that are added to foods to enhance flavor or texture, and they end up confusing our taste buds, turning us toward the addictive path of empty promises.

Eating MSG?

IF IT'S IN A BOX, YOU PROBABLY ARE!

The secret ingredient in a famous fried-chicken recipe is MSG (monosodium glutamate), a flavor-enhancing chemical compound, which provides a savory taste to food. In 1959, the FDA classified MSG as a food additive "generally recognized as safe." MSG is a widely used additive in the food industry, but you may not find it listed as an ingredient. Even products that claim "no MSG" on their labels may, in fact, contain MSG. It can be hidden under the heading of natural flavors, hydrolyzed protein, or vegetable stock, for instance.

While the U.S. government currently has no restrictions or warnings on MSG, numerous scientists from around the world have repeatedly confirmed that MSG causes a range of health problems, including obesity.

As an example, researchers at the University of North Carolina at Chapel Hill, working with Chinese researchers, published a study in 2008 that found a positive link between MSG intake and obesity: the prevalence of being overweight was significantly higher in MSG users than in non-users.

Addicted to fake sugar?
DITCH THE DIET DRINKS!

Aspartame is a synthetic sweetener used in most diet drinks. It is also the ingredient in those little packets of NutraSweet or Equal. Aspartame is known to change the brain's chemistry, causing seizures, neurological diseases, birth defects, memory loss, vertigo, depression, phobias, ADD, anxiety attacks, blindness, decreased vision, high blood pressure, fibromyalgia, lymphoma, and many other known and as yet to be known disorders. Aspartame poisoning can even mimic the symptoms of multiple sclerosis.

Janet Starr Hull, creator of the *Aspartame Detox Program*, calls aspartame "sweet poison." She states, "the dangers of aspartame poisoning have been a well-guarded secret since the 1980s. The research and history of aspartame is conclusive as a cause of illness and toxic reactions in the human body. Side effects can occur gradually, can be immediate, or can be acute reactions. It is a dangerous chemical food additive, and its use during pregnancy and by children is one of the greatest modern tragedies of all."

According to Lendon Smith, MD, an enormous segment of the population suffers from side effects associated with aspartame. There are users who do not appear to suffer immediate reactions, but all are potentially susceptible to the long-term damage caused by excitatory amino acids, phenylalanine, methanol, and diketopiperazine (DKP)—the toxic by-products of aspartame. And there are numerous potential deleterious effects, including seizures, blindness and aggression. In fact, Theresa Dale, ND, author of *Revitalize Your Hormones* and founder of The Wellness and Anti-Aging Research Center, confirms that there are over 92 different health symptoms at the root of modern disease for which aspartame can be the causative factor.

Now that you know how sick it can make you are you still wondering if it can really make you fat? Already in 2005, a University of Texas study linked aspartame-sweetened diet drinks with increased obesity. Even though aspartame can boast ZERO calories, there are several ways in which it actually increases weight gain and unsightliness:

- It overloads the liver with toxicity, causing excess fat to build up inside the liver. This is referred to as "fatty liver." When the liver is compromised, it is difficult to lose weight.
- It causes fluid retention, cellulite, and a bloated and puffy appearance.
- It creates unstable blood-sugar levels, which increases the appetite and causes food cravings.
- It suppresses production of serotonin, thereby increasing the specific craving for empty-calorie, high-carbohydrate foods.
- It is a drug that affects the dopamine system of the brain, creating an addictive cycle of unhealthy eating choices.

Want to ditch suffering and weight gain? Then *begin* by ditching empty-calorie foods loaded with toxic chemicals, such as aspartame, once and for all!

Fake Fat Makes You Fatter!

Junk-food manufacturers have been sensitive to the rumors that their foods make people fat. So to solve the problem of empty calories and high fat content, they have created fake, zero-calorie sweeteners and fake fat!

There are reasons to avoid excessive fat, not the least being that many of the toxic chemicals that end up in our food are stored in the fatty cells of animals and fish, in cream and butter, and in vegetable oils. But there are also powerful reasons to avoid the fake fats. It turns out that like the fake sweeteners, fake fats also make you fat!

In 1996, the FDA approved *Olestra* (brand name *Olean*) as a replacement for fats and oils in snack foods. Since then it has had its ups and downs but is still used for some light or fat-free snacks.

Olestra is a kind of fat that is indigestible, so it just moves through the body and out the other end. However, it can pick up a few things as it moves along, including fat-soluble nutrients.

It turns out that not only is this fake fat empty, but it also siphons out important fat-soluble nutrients that are already in the internal environment, especially the *carotenoids*.

Carotenoids include lutein, beta-carotene, and lycopene, and are a valuable antioxidant. It also grabs hold of the fat-soluble vitamins A, D, E, and K and escorts them out of the body. Other fat-soluble phytonutrients may be at risk as well.

Several studies were done on the carotenoid-depleting effects of olestra. In one study, the equivalent of sixteen olestra-based, fat-free Pringles chips a day for two weeks depleted lutein levels in the blood by 20%. Further, the equivalent of six chips a day for four weeks depleted lycopene levels in the blood by 40%.

Finally, is the issue of how olestra makes you fat! A study published in *Behavioral Neuroscience* in 2011 clearly showed a correlation between olestra and weight gain in rats. Rats fed a high-fat diet supplemented with fat-free Pringles potato chips gained more weight than those supplemented with regular, high-fat Pringles.

Researchers theorized that when the "sensory signals that a high-calorie meal is about to be consumed is not followed by the anticipated high number of calories, this 'degrades' the link between sensory signals and the learned control of energy regulation." This means that "empty promises" confuse the body.

The Hidden Truth about GMOs
WHAT MANUFACTURERS AREN'T TELLING YOU!

When it comes to processed foods, GMOs can hide in all kinds of things. Which of these would you guess is likely made of GMOs?

Hydrolyzed vegetable protein	Ascorbic acid
Hydrogenated starch	Citric acid
Baking powder	Inositol
Sorbitol	

If you guessed all of them, you were right!

According to the Grocery Manufacturers Association, an estimated 80% of processed foods sold in the United States contain ingredients that have been genetically modified. Sadly, most Americans are unaware of this. Federal regulatory officials continue to disregard GMO concerns and stonewall all efforts to mandate proper GMO labeling.

Michael Pollan, a leading writer on food policy, said in a recent interview on GMO technology, "The real benefit of GM [Genetic Modification] to these companies is really the ability to control the genetic resources on which humankind depends…It represents a whole new level of corporate control over our food supply—a handful of companies are owning the seeds, controlling the farmers and controlling our choices." This is the *Brave New World** of our food supply. Eating GMOs is not good for us, for the earth, or it turns out for the protection of our freedoms.

If you want to make a difference, please join the fight for labeling of GMOs. If we don't know what we're buying, how can we be free to choose what we are feeding into our internal environment?

THE LAKE ERIE SYNDROME

Organic sources of phosphate found in meat, eggs, dairy, grains, beans, and nuts are enough to tip the scales from health to disease in the modern omnivore diet. So imagine what happens when we add inorganic sources of phosphate in the form of food additives!

Many processed foods contain phosphate-based additives. Look for terms such as phosphate or phosphoric in the ingredients list. Then, there are also phosphate-based additives that are not immediately obvious from the name.

Phosphates can be found in preservatives, emulsifiers, stabilizers, thickeners, self-raising flours, soda and cola drinks—and that's just the beginning. Eating a diet high in processed foods assures that you are experiencing extremely elevated levels of phosphates in your system.

Hertha Hafer, author of *The Hidden Drug: Dietary Phosphate*, makes the connection:

> Today it is known that phosphate run off from cleaning products, fertilizers and agrichemicals has a highly damaging effect on the earth's ecosystems. Environmentally concerned people across the world very quickly instigated successful programs to protect plants, tributaries, marine life, and so forth. In contrast, few people realize that phosphate-rich foods and beverages pose an equally serious health hazard to sensitive children and adults.

Brave New World by author Aldous Huxley is a fiction novel about a futuristic society based on pleasure without moral repercussions.

Toxic, inorganic phosphates can be found in everything from vaccines, children's vitamins, infant formulas, drugs and clothing, to the air we breathe on airplanes. The inorganic phosphates that permeate our food and medical system, and our way of life are especially problematic for those who are already compromised by neurological syndromes, weakened immune systems, and a heightened sensitivity to phosphates.

There are also the unlisted ingredients in the foods we buy. Paula Baillie-Hamilton, MD, says in her book *The Body Restoration Plan*:

> The organophosphates were initially developed for use in human warfare... However, what really struck me about organophosphates was that this same group of chemicals had a commercial use: to fatten up livestock!...What made it even worse was that the same type of chemical used to fatten up cattle (at very low doses) was also found on our food (again in very low doses) as a crop insecticide.

Another compelling reason to buy organic!

CAN YOU AFFORD TO BE A JUNKIVORE?

When inflation is accounted for, we spend about 1.3 times more on food per person than we did 50 years ago. Real food costs have gone up. But when you look at the empty calories of the "food" in a junkivore's shopping cart, what are we really getting for the money? Let's take a look at a day in the life of a junkivore.

A Day in the Life of a Junkivore

Groggy awakening—you grab a bag of Hostess Sweet Sixteen donuts and a cold Starbucks Coffee Flavor frappe from the fridge to gulp down on the way to work

✓ You've just started your day ingesting over 40 toxic substances.

Late morning blood-sugar slump and hunger pangs are assuaged by chewing a couple pieces of Orbit Wildberry Remix Sugarfree gum.

✓ You've just ingested more than 17 toxic products, including aspartame.

Lunch is a can of Pepsi from the vending machine, a bag of Frito-Lay Salsa with Queso Cheetos, and a Sub (sandwich) with cold cuts from the deli case at a commercial grocery store.

✓ Whoa! The deli sandwich alone contains over 49 toxic products. In total, you've ingested over 89 different chemical toxins in your lunch.

By late afternoon, there's some brain fog. How about a candy bar?

✓ You've just ingested another 12 plus toxic substances.

For supper, something easy: Boil spaghetti; open a can of Del Monte Meat-flavored Pasta sauce, and put some deli garlic bread in the toaster oven.

✓ You're feasting on at least 38 toxic products.

Add some grated Parmesan cheese from a box (processed) to improve the garlic bread and sprinkle it over the spaghetti with meat sauce.

✓ You've just added 4 more toxins!

Feeling guilty about not eating veggies, so grab some Birds Eye Steamed Fresh Mixed frozen vegetables from the freezer compartment, pour some in a little bowl, and stick it in the microwave oven. (While no toxic substances are listed in the ingredients, consider the residual pesticides, free radicals, and other toxins from the microwave heating, and nutrient loss of the food.)

Late evening and time to relax—or should I say crash? Too exhausted to do anything more than watch some TV before sleeping. But TV calls for munchies, so how about some microwave popcorn?

✓ Add another 4 or more toxic ingredients, including a big dose of trans fats!

It is hard to tell how many more toxic chemicals may lurk under the headings of things like natural and artificial flavors. Other unlisted ingredients on this menu: salt may come with dextrose, potassium iodine, and aluminum additives; salt, bread and processed or shredded cheeses may also contain aluminum additives.

The junkivore menu cost: $11.60
Total calories: 3006, total protein: 79 grams

Junkivores are meat-eating chemivores who have devolved to the next level of a degraded diet. Sadly, many vegetarians and even some vegans have also fallen into a denatured, acid-based junkivore diet. The *Urban Dictionary* defines the term *junkitarian* as someone who is technically a vegetarian in that they abstain from meat, but who negates all the potential health benefits by eating mostly junk food.

This is why some of the vegetarians I have consulted with in the past are just as acidic and sick as those who eat meat. In short, they are junkitarians and not true vegetarians.

A true vegetarian should be defined as *someone who eats vegetation* (whole plant foods), not someone who eats a diet that includes processed foods, even if that food comes from health food stores and carries an organic label.

This is why I wanted to come up with a new name for myself that would honestly describe the type of diet I was eating. So I did! I now call myself an *ecotarian!*

People sometimes tell me that they would love to be an ecotarian and eat the kind of diet I eat, but they just cannot afford it. Is it true that it costs more to eat well? I really wanted to know for myself, so let's take a look at a day in the life of an ecotarian—one who eats for the sustainability of their body and planet.

A Day in the Life of an Ecotarian

You would enjoy a half-hour walk, jog, or yoga; a quart of purified water; some deep breathing; and a few minutes in the sun, followed by an Apple-Ginger-Kale smoothie (apple, small ginger thumb, lemon, kale).

For lunch, how about quick and easy lettuce wraps with lots of fruit salsa? The salsa can be made up ahead and kept in the fridge for quick meals or snacking. Add a glass of Clean, Green, and Lean (spinach, lettuce, celery, cucumber, and kale for an alkalizing boost!

A mid-afternoon snack of a Berry Good Smoothie provides an antioxidant boost.

For supper, a Watercress-Papaya Salad of luscious greens, Vidalia onion, and papaya, with Sweet and Sour Oil-Free Dressing.

The ecotarian menu cost: $13.77

Total calories: 1985, total protein: 69 grams

The FDA recommends 65 grams of protein a day for people consuming 2000 calories and 80 grams a day for those consuming 2500. From this, we can see that the ecotarian menu is right on with 69 grams, *and* it is food without chemicals from natural sources!

As you can see, I pulled out all the stops to provide you with a highly nourishing, varied, delicious, gourmet menu. It turns out the ecotarian menu costs $2.17 more, or 15% more than the junkivore menu.

To make the ecotarian diet even less expensive than the junkivore diet, here are some tips for eco living:

✓ For those of you with a green thumb, grow your own backyard garden. This is by far the best way to cut down on food costs through the growing season.

✓ Get a hydroponic growing system like the Tower Garden for your terrace or rooftop. It will pay for itself and more over time.

✓ Consider planting your own fruit trees. You'll have more than you can eat once the fruit comes on, so have fun making exchanges with your neighbors.

✓ Shop at the local farmer's market. Here's a tip: You'll find the freshest produce and the best items in the first ½ hour of the market, but you may also find great deals at the end of the market from farmers who don't want to take produce back home with them.

✓ Buy in bulk through a local food coop or an online buying club like *Green Polka Box*. You'll be able to find some food items online for much less than what you would pay at the health food or grocery store.

Let's Talk About *Real* Costs

JUNKIVORE DIET

High calorie

Highly processed, denatured foods

A few synthetic vitamins

Feeds food addiction

Paves the way to ecological breakdown

Loaded with chemicals and GMO
    ingredients

ECOTARIAN DIET

Low calorie

Whole foods

A cornucopia of phytonutrients

Just real, living food

Nourishes the body

Promotes a healthy internal
    environment

The *real* cost of a junkivore diet eventually includes the cost of medical intervention—drugs, surgeries, and other aspects of conventional disease management. Medical bills are the cause of more than 60% of all bankruptcy filings in the United States.

So really, can you afford to be a junkivore?

DIETARY DEVOLUTION #4
FROM JUNKIVORE TO DRUGIVORE

The junkivore diet is already nearly drug-like, in that it is more about feeding chemical addictions than nourishing our cellular environment. In the final degenerative cycle of dietary devolution, drugs begin to take the place of missing nutrients as the foundation of bodily functions, mental health, and immunity.

Today, we live in a war-like mentality such as the war against cancer and the war against bugs. We spend billions of dollars each year on research investigating *the cure* but generally speaking, never *the cause*. Every year, around wintertime, we are encouraged to get a flu shot to help ward off an attacker "bug," never to be told that the wintertime flu can generally be avoided if we don't overeat during the holidays, or at least juice fasted for a few days to remove the accumulated, undigested waste that feed the "bugs."

Similar to using pesticides on a sick plant to kill the "bugs," drugs like "antibiotics" are used to kill the "germs" and, generally, to our detriment.

Drugs including flu shots, immunizations, and antibiotics have a powerfully debilitating effect on the trillions of organisms that populate our internal environment. You might say that within us, on a microscopic level, there is a landscape, an internal terrain, as amazing as that of the earth, or even the universe, and inhabitants who are either beneficial or not.

To think of my internal environment as a living, breathing, densely populated universe astounds me.

Did you know?

There are at least ten times as many bacteria in the human body as cells.

Even the mitochondria, the power plants of our cells, may have evolved from a symbiotic relationship with free-living bacteria.

Unfortunately, drugs wipe out our microbial populations and, to make matters worse, trigger the mutation of extremely harmful superbugs.

Another consideration is the side effects of drugs. Have you ever heard them listed in TV commercials? Pretty scary, and yet people still take them!

In 1982, Dr. Bernard Jensen wrote:

> The United States Department of Health, Education and Welfare's Task Force on Drug Prescriptions has reported that physicians tend to over-prescribe medicines, both in quantity and variety, for the same illness. About 300,000 people in this country are hospitalized each year for severe adverse drug reactions. Approximately 18,000 die annually from side effects of [prescription] drugs. Many patients become ill from medications without getting any benefit from them.

Only ten years later, those figures are shockingly higher: More than 1.8 million Americans suffered serious, toxic side effects from medical drugs, and had to be hospitalized. By 1996, those figures were averaging over two million Americans a year! Additionally, one-third of those admissions were due to the toxic effects of medications. In 1996, it was reported that nearly 700,000 Americans die each year of secondary side effects from medications. As you can see, pharmaceutical drugs are more dangerous than you might believe.

Ultimately, drugs affect our internal landscape by:

- creating other diseases they call side effects;
- making war on the complex web of living organisms and organic structures that make up our metabolism;
- decreasing the biodiversity of bacteria in the intestinal tract;
- destroying the acid/alkaline balance, oxygenation and hydration of the internal landscape;
- polluting our fluid systems, leading to further degeneration of the nervous system and organs;
- reducing sexual function and fertility;
- directly poisoning and killing us. Prescription drugs are one of the leading causes of death in the U.S.;
- chronically weakening our lives and those of animals through water supplies that are contaminated by trace amounts of numerous drugs;
- triggering the mutation of destructive superbugs, aggressive reducer organisms immune to our medical weapons.

Drugs are part of a medical industry in which diseases are no longer cured, but rather managed. Mainstream internal medicine is not about restoring the health of the internal landscape (as in the days of Hippocrates), it is about annihilating microbes through chemical intervention.

While drugs may force a particular effect, such as lowering blood pressure, they ultimately disrupt the ecological equilibrium of the body further. All synthetic drugs, including synthetic vitamins, are extremely acidifying to the body. This is why one drug often leads to another, and another, as ecological breakdowns are accelerated until finally you're taking a handful of drugs with every meal. Look into the medicine cabinet of an elderly person and you'll see what I mean!

THE DEVOLUTION OF DISEASE

A powerful research paper called *Disease in Human Evolution* (1996) describes how historical changes in lifestyle and landscape created conditions for new diseases and epidemics within human populations. Major changes took place with the Agricultural Revolution. In conjunction with the shift to an acidifying diet, cities sprang up, creating the conditions for infectious epidemics and widespread diseases of malnutrition.

In the last century, among populations in developed and developing nations, infectious disease declined while chronic degenerative diseases rose dramatically. Now, we are on the cusp of a third epidemiological transition, a reemergence of infectious disease that is antibiotic resistant and transmitted on a global scale.

We are now living in a new world of a degraded environment, inside and out. We are vulnerable to new, drug-resistant varieties of infectious disease and never-before-seen infectious diseases. You could say that we are taking infectious disease to a new level.

In previous centuries, epidemic infectious diseases were local or regional in nature. Now, with air travel, a new disease can spread around the globe within days. Most of the following conditions could be called cultural disease vectors since they have to do with human society, industry and business strategies.

Some of them that have the potential to breed infectious disease throughout our world and completely redefine how we live (and possibly *if* we live), and include:

- the crossing of pathogens between species (mad-cow disease, for example);
- the destruction and pollution of natural ecosystems;
- the problems of dense population centers;
- elevated levels of nuclear radiation, and the proliferation of nuclear arms;
- the spreading of GMOs;
- micro-biotic adaptation (drug and pesticide resistance);
- the morphing of micro-biota to pathological forms within the degraded environment of our internal landscape.

This has been a grand overview of the current state of our food affairs. Perhaps we could say, like Charles Dickens said of his own times, "It was the best of times, it was the worst of times."

Bruce Lipton says, "Crisis ignites evolution." But evolution involves critical junctures of sudden change that we could call revolution—an action that sparks evolving back to "what once was"—a toxic-free, "green" planet and a toxic-free, "green" body! Thus, the first step toward changing our planet's environmental crisis is to become an internal environmentalist. So, join hands with me in the *Ecotarian Revolution*, and be the change we want to see in the world!!

Chapter 7

HAS YOUR BODY BEEN SENDING YOU AN S-O-S SIGNAL?

Pain and suffering are your body's S-O-S signals, attempting to get your attention to "Answer the Call" of change!

If your diet falls somewhere on the scale of dietary devolution, the prospect of breaking all your old habits may seem overwhelming. Let's face it—change is not always easy. Old habits that have been ingrained in us since childhood can be very strong and are not so easy to break, especially when it comes to food. So unless you have life-threatening health issue, you can take more time in making the shift. Returning to the original frugivore diet that you were designed for involves not only moving into a whole new lifestyle, but also eliminating some staples from your old diet. For most, it is hard to know where to begin, so I've created a simple plan.

To begin your restoration, you must heed your body's S-O-S signal and stop burning the wrong type of salt, oil, and sugar into your internal environment!

S-O-S

Start your move up the alkaline scale by eliminating the wrong type of salt, oil and sugar, and replacing them with the right type of salt, oil, and sugar. That is just eliminating three things, but these three things will make such a huge difference. This is because approximately 99% of all processed foods are loaded with highly refined salt, oil, and sugar. And these ingredients are among the top three acidifiers that drive the oxygen out of your internal environment.

Salt, oil, and sugar tend to show up in foods that are full of other toxic chemical additives, too. So when you eliminate and replace these three toxic ingredients, you'll avoid almost every acidic, oxygen-depleting, eco-destroying food on the market.

Your *Ecotarian Revolution* has begun!

THE WRONG TYPE OF SALT

If the salt (or the processed food that contains it) in your pantry has been refined, throw it out! The wrong type of salt to your cells is like too much sunlight to a grape. While salt is essential for life, the wrong type of salt dehydrates your cells and lowers their electrical potential, which is like running down the stored energy of a battery. This lowers the bio-electric energy available to our body's cells for the purposes of achieving homeostasis, and a state of optimal health and well-being.

There's an enormous difference between the refined salt most people are accustomed to and a whole-food salt. Refined table salt is actually 97.5% sodium chloride and 2.5% chemicals such as moisture absorbents, anti-caking agents and possibly an iodine-containing compound.

Dried at over 1,200°F, the excessive heat substantially alters the natural chemical structure of the salt, regardless of whether it is land salt or sea salt. What remains after most salts are chemically cleaned is a degraded structure of sodium chloride, a form of salt that your body identifies as something unnatural.

Deposits of salt contain iodine and other trace minerals. Through the process of refinement, however, the natural web of mineral nutrients is lost, so one of them—iodine—in the form of potassium iodide, is added back in. Essential trace minerals, removed as impurities, are replaced with anti-caking agents such as aluminum hydroxide, sodium aluminosilicate, or other chemical names you can't pronounce. Salt is also processed with aluminum, so aluminum toxicity over a lifetime of ingestion is a real issue. While our water systems are fluoridated, in Europe, salt is fluoridated.

These various forms of unnatural salt have earned the name "white poison."

As for iodine, there is a reason for adding it back to salt. An oft-quoted talk by UNICEF Deputy Director Kul Gautam to an American Thyroid Association Symposium in 2007 included the following:

> Even a moderate [iodine] deficiency, especially in pregnant women and infants, lowers their intelligence by 10 to 15 IQ points, with incalculable damage to social and economic development of nations and communities. Today, over one billion people in the world suffer from iodine deficiency, and 38 million babies born every year are not protected from brain damage due to iodine deficiency.

Now, with levels of radiation increasing in large parts of the world, getting enough iodine to protect the thyroid is also a grave issue. If you hold the belief that at least you are getting iodine from refined salt, keep in mind that virtually none of the salt in processed foods is iodized.

The body isolates excess or bio-unavailable salt by extracting water from your cells to neutralize it. The resulting consequence is a less-than-ideal fluid equilibrium. For every gram of sodium chloride your body cannot get rid of, 23 times that amount of cell water is used to neutralize the salt. Thus, refined salt causes excess fluid buildup around the cells, which can contribute to unsightly cellulite, along with rheumatism, arthritis, gout, kidney stones, and gallstones. These types of salt are inorganic, which means the body doesn't identify it as "real food," but rather as a poison.

Regrettably, refined salt not only sits on most every kitchen table across our nation, it is found in almost every processed product that you eat. When you consider that the average person consumes 4,000 to 6,000 milligrams of sodium chloride each day, and heavy users can ingest as much as 10,000 milligrams in a day, it is clear that this is a serious and pervasive issue.

Researchers and physicians around the world have found that a diet high in salt contributes to a number of health risks, such as high blood pressure, heart disease, stroke, and certain kinds of cancers. Still, the right kind of salt is as fundamental to our life as air and water, and without it we could not exist.

THE RIGHT TYPE OF SALT

The ultimate whole-food salt is found in vegetables like celery. Unlike many other vegetables, celery is relatively high in natural sodium. In fact, the average stalk of celery contains about 35 mg of sodium, but unlike inorganic, rock-based sodium chloride in table salt, the sodium in celery is in a chelated, organic form. Turning inorganic minerals into organic minerals takes place through the power of microbial action in the soil. Plants take in the "digested" minerals from the soil and convert them into a form that we can use—in effect, turning rocks into food.

However, all table salts are not the same. While I believe vegetables such as celery are the best way for us to consume adequate amounts of sodium every day, for those who add salt to their food, the brand I recommend is Celtic sea salt®.

Celtic sea salt is harvested off the coast of France using methods originating with the Celts many centuries ago, leaving it in its natural crystalline form. The natural methods used to harvest this particular brand of sea salt enable the crystals to maintain a wonderful, clean flavor. The diverse array of minerals craved by the human body remains inherent within the salt as well.

Celtic sea salt imparts a pure, fresh taste to your meals, rather than the harsh flavor of regular table salt. But more importantly, nearly eighty vital mineral electrolytes are found in the tiny, gray crystals of Celtic sea salt. This whole salt will give you energy, and promote healthy body functions such as immune system strengthening and the absorption of nutritious elements from food.

The trace minerals play an important part in cleansing the body and aiding in healthy digestion. Many health-care practitioners like myself include Celtic sea salt in their regular diet, as the balance of minerals and nutrients is an optimum choice for those living a healthy lifestyle.

Unlike refined table salt, Celtic sea salt helps:

- regulate water balance throughout the body.
- promote a healthy pH balance in the cells (particularly your brain cells).
- promote a healthy blood sugar.
- reduce signs of aging.

- assist in the generation of hydroelectric energy in the cells.
- with absorption of food particles throughout the intestinal tract.
- support respiratory health.
- promote sinus health.
- prevent muscle cramps.
- promote bone strength.
- regulate sleep patterns.
- support libido.
- promote vascular health.
- regulate blood pressure.

THE WRONG TYPE OF OIL

If you have polyunsaturated vegetable oils (or processed foods that contain them) in your pantry, throw 'em out! These are the oils that remain liquid even in the refrigerator. Consuming the wrong type of oil is like dumping petroleum into the earth's tributaries. While fats and oils are essential for life, the wrong type clogs your cells, lowers their electrical potential, impedes the flow of oxygen, creates insulin resistance, and can cause a chain reaction of free-radical damage (explained below) and ultimately a weakened immune system.

While every whole plant food contains a certain amount of fats, calories, carbohydrates and proteins, the problem begins with extracting a particular part, such as oil, from the whole. Dr. Caldwell Esselstyn's studies at the renowned Cleveland Clinic demonstrated that any type of processed, extracted oil could, over time, leave a sticky plaque buildup in the arteries and veins that inhibits blood flow. However, mounting evidence reveals that polyunsaturated vegetable oils, generally thought of as healthy, may be the most harmful of all extracted oils.

Polyunsaturated vegetable oils are the wrong type of oil.

A glaze of polyunsaturated oils in your internal environment can contribute to the risk of degenerative diseases, including cancer. One of the reasons for this is that polyunsaturated oils turn rancid more quickly than other oils. In fact, flaxseed oil, the most highly touted oil in the health industry, is known to become rancid within a few hours after it has been pressed. This makes polyunsaturated oils the wrong type of oil even if they are organic, cold-pressed and unrefined.

The acidity of oils cannot be measured by the use of pH paper, but they can be measured through laboratory methods such as titration. The acid value of oil is a measure of its rancidity.

Rancidity is a chemical change in oil produced by oxidation—the reaction of oxygen from the air with the unsaturated fatty acids in the oil. The oxidation process speeds up over time, so the longer the oil sits around, the more rancid it becomes.

Another concern with polyunsaturated oils is that the ratio between omega-3 and omega-6 fatty acids is imbalanced. A properly balanced ratio of omega-6 to omega-3 fatty acids allows the body, in part, to maintain a healthy response to inflammation. The imbalance is worsened when manufacturers remove the omega-3 fatty acids in refining vegetable oils (to increase shelf-life), leaving only the omega-6 portion of the fatty acids intact. The excess of omega-6 fatty acids contributes, then, to inflammation, a fatty liver, metabolic syndrome, obesity, and weakened immunity.

In the case of oil, saturation means that at the molecular level, it is saturated with hydrogen atoms. When oils are polyunsaturated, this means that some hydrogen atoms have been removed, which opens the structure of the molecule in a way that makes it more vulnerable to attack by free radicals. Dr. Ray Peat explains, "When unsaturated oils are exposed to free radicals they can create chain reactions of free radicals that spread the damage in the cell, and contribute to the cell's aging." The mitochondria—the aerobic energy factories of the cell—are especially vulnerable to free radical damage.

Free radicals can arise spontaneously from within our internal environment in response to various stresses. We can also bring them into our bodies by ingesting the wrong kinds of oil, by exposing ourselves to radioactive fall-out, or by inhaling diesel exhaust or cigarette smoke, for instance.

The research Dr. Peat has drawn together indicates some sobering facts:

- Polyunsaturated oils weaken the immune system's function in ways that are similar to the damage caused by radiation, hormone imbalance, cancer, aging, or viral infections.

- Cancer cannot occur, unless there are unsaturated oils in the diet.
- Alcoholic cirrhosis of the liver cannot occur unless there are unsaturated oils in the diet.
- Heart disease can be produced by unsaturated oils.
- Polyunsaturated oils can contribute to the risk of arthritis, diabetes, heart disease and accelerated aging.

Polyunsaturated oils to avoid include soybean, corn, canola, cottonseed, safflower, sesame, grapeseed, almond and most other vegetable and nut oils. The first four listed (soybean, corn, canola, and cottonseed) are commonly extracted from genetically modified crops (GMOs), which makes them doubly dangerous.

Trans fats are the wrong type of fat.

Trans fats are created through partial hydrogenation. Hydrogenation is the process by which hydrogen is forced into highly heated vegetable oil. Partially hydrogenating oils creates a softer texture, making it the perfect consistency for items such as margarine and imitation whipped cream. When oils are partially hydrogenated, the molecules form trans configurations, which means they have an odd shape for fat molecules.

Oils and fats are essentially the same thing, the main difference being that oils are liquid at room temperature while fats are solid. Trans fats, however, are the most harmful fats to your arteries and are known to create cardiovascular disease. These unhealthy fats are often found in fast foods such as fried chicken and French fries; junk foods such as doughnuts, cookies, candy bars, potato chips, pastries, and crackers; and in processed staples on the grocery shelves, from soup mixes to margarine.

Like the polyunsaturated fats from which they are derived, trans fats are known to cause intense free-radical activity, which can turn cell membranes rancid and stiff. The resulting rigidity impedes the free flow of oxygen through the membrane and interrupts electronic transfers of energy, producing a kind of bioelectrical short. Trans fats also interfere with the circulation of oxygen in the blood, creating a state of acidosis.

Be aware: according to FDA guidelines, products containing less than 0.5 grams of trans fat per serving can list zero grams trans fat on their nutritional labels! As a result, an 8-serving bag of chips with "zero grams trans fat" may, in fact, contain as much as 4 grams of trans fat. If partially hydrogenated oil is listed as an ingredient, there are trans fats.

Lard is the wrong type of fat.

Lard (pig fat) is usually referred to as a saturated fat, but when pigs are fed the standard diet of corn and soybeans, their meat (pork) becomes higher in polyunsaturated fat (around 32%) and pretty much all of that is omega-6.

Paul Jaminet, a scientist and co-author of *The Perfect Health Diet,* tells us that traditional diets fed to pigs in past generations would have kept the percentage of polyunsaturated fat in pork between three and 9%, but industrialized farming has changed that. As you might imagine, the same thing occurs in the fats of other omnivores and herbivores that are fed an unnatural diet of almost exclusively grains and beans.

THE RIGHT TYPE OF OIL

For the right type of oil, eat fats and oils in the form of a whole food—do not extract them. Extracted oils are not a whole food! They are 100% fat! Whole-food fats and oils include avocados, coconuts, olives, nuts, and seeds.

However, if you choose to use extracted oils, think olive oil or tropical oils like coconut and macadamia nut oil. Tropical oils, which are soft or solid at room temperature, are saturated. They are stable at higher temperatures, so they don't become rancid in our tissues, like the seed oils from plants grown in colder climates do. At the molecular level, it means that the oil is naturally saturated with hydrogen atoms.

In the past, we heard a lot about saturated fat and its bad effect on cholesterol levels. Yet, according to neurobiologist Stephan Guyenet, more and more evidence is accumulating to indicate an absence of association between saturated fat intake and cholesterol or heart-attack risk. Saturated fats are emerging as the better choice.

When we eat relatively more saturated fat, it inhibits the
potential damage of the unsaturated fat that we eat.

Coconut oil is a saturated fat that contains medium-chain fatty acids, which have some great benefits. It has been shown to improve thyroid function, lower cholesterol, and protect from heart disease and cancer. Coconut oil is unique in its ability to prevent weight-gain and promote weight loss by increasing the metabolic rate. So if you need to use extracted oil, think coconut oil!

Or consider monounsaturated oils like olive or macadamia nut oil. Monounsaturated oils are more stable than polyunsaturated oils. While monounsaturated vegetables oils have a certain amount of polyunsaturated oil as part of their composition, olive oil, for instance, only contains 11%.

The high ratio of monounsaturated oil keeps the polyunsaturated component of the oil stabilized. So, if you're going to use the monounsaturated oils:

- look for high quality (extra-virgin), cold-pressed, organic oils;
- choose oils that are in a dark, glass bottle;
- store them in a cool, dark place;
- don't overheat in cooking; and
- use sparingly.

Olive oil may last up to a year, with optimal storage. Still, do the sniff test when you open the bottle and if there's any question of rancidity, DO NOT USE!

Checking for rancidity also extends to products that contain oils, fats, whole grains, or nuts and seeds. You may need to establish new kitchen practices to accommodate faster spoilage of whole foods as you move into a whole food *EcoDiet* lifestyle.

- Purchase oils, whole grains, nuts and seeds, or products containing them, in small quantities, and eat them within a short time.
- Store oils in a cool, dark cabinet or in the refrigerator.
- Store nuts and whole-grain flours in the freezer.

What about omega-3 fatty acids? Here's the conundrum: omega-3 and omega-6 fatty acids are found in polyunsaturated oils—the wrong oils! While the omega-3 and omega-6 fatty acids are "essential," the body is actually able to produce them. This fact has been scientifically documented as far back as the 1940s.

The problem is that the typical American diet contains excessive amounts of omega-6, to our detriment. Recommendations for optimum ratios of these fatty acids vary. However, one thing everyone agrees on is that most of us are not getting enough omega-3 from our diet to balance the excessive load of omega-6. Omega-3s are contained in many fruits, vegetables and seeds like chia and flax, as well as walnuts.

The greatest issue is the elimination of refined, polyunsaturated,
omega-6 oils and the processed foods that contain them!

Once you eliminate the wrong oils, the fatty-acid ratio will naturally begin to balance itself. You'll also find high ratios of whole-food omega-3 fats in seeds and nuts like walnuts, brazil nuts, and flax seed; vegetables like spinach, kale, broccoli, cauliflower, and brussel sprouts; herbs and spices like basil, oregano, marjoram, and mustard seeds; and fruits like avocados and strawberries.

A low-fat, whole-fat *EcoDiet* is the key to promoting a clean, green, sustainable internal environment.

THE WRONG TYPE OF SUGAR

If the sugar (or the processed food that contains it) in your pantry has been refined, throw it out! The wrong type of sugar to your cells is like pouring espresso into the gas tank of your automobile. While sugar from fruits is essential for life, the wrong type of sugar may get your energy temporarily revved up, but shortly, you will crash and burn!

Processed, refined white sugar, the table sugar that most people use every day, is harmful to your health, even in small amounts. It is another form of "white poison," and it only got worse with the advent of GMO sugar beets.

Dr. Robert Lustig is a specialist on pediatric hormone disorders and the leading expert in childhood obesity at the University of California, San Francisco School of Medicine, one of the best medical schools in the country. He published his first paper on childhood obesity approximately 12 years ago, and he has been treating patients and doing research on the disorder ever since. He says that our nation's excessive consumption of sugar is the primary reason for the skyrocketing numbers of obese and diabetic Americans in the past 30 years.

The average person consumes 150 pounds of sugar per year compared to just 7½ pounds consumed on average in the year 1700.

—Mehmet Oz, MD

This is 30 times more than our grandparents! Until the 1970s, most of the sugar we ate came from sucrose, which is derived from sugar beets or sugar cane. After that, sugars manufactured from corn, such as corn syrup, fructose, dextrose, dextrin, and especially high fructose corn syrup, began to gain popularity as sweeteners because they were much less expensive to produce. High fructose corn syrup is one of our worse dietary enemies and should be avoided at all costs.

High fructose corn syrup can be manipulated to contain equal amounts of fructose and glucose, or up to 80% fructose and 20% glucose. With almost four times the fructose, high fructose corn syrup delivers a double danger compared to refined white sugar, and it's found in almost every processed food that sits on your grocer's shelves.

Not only is high fructose corn syrup considered one of the major contributors to obesity and Type 2 diabetes, a study published in *Environmental Health* (2009) reported that high fructose corn syrup was commonly tainted with mercury and that traces of mercury were found in many processed foods. The mercury appears to come from caustic soda and hydrochloric acid, two chemicals used in the manufacture of high fructose corn syrup that can, depending on their manufacturing process, contain trace amounts of mercury.

Other sweeteners derived from corn include the sugar alcohols, among them malitol, sorbitol, xylitol, and erythritol. These sweeteners are created through a fermentation process. Corn sweeteners are often made with GMO corn; so, if you want to avoid GMOs, avoid corn-derived sweeteners.

Another dietary enemy is synthetic sugar such as aspartame (marketed as NutraSweet®, Equal®, and Spoonful®). It should be avoided at all costs. When the temperature of aspartame exceeds 86°F, which is most likely to occur during shipping in warm parts of the country or times of the year, it converts to formaldehyde and then to formic acid, which causes metabolic acidosis. This means that the pH imbalance is systemic and severe enough that the body no longer has the ability to effectively neutralize the acidic condition.

THE RIGHT TYPE OF SUGAR

Naturally occurring sugars in whole-food form such as fruits, berries, raw cane, and vegetables can be healthful. These sugars naturally support your pancreas and your brain and boost your immunity, build and tone your muscles, and can even assist you in losing weight. For example, complex sugars found in goji berries, have been clinically shown to alkalize your environment, maintain youthfulness and increase longevity, break down tumors, improve eyesight, combat free radicals, strengthen the liver and pancreas, boost your metabolism, and promote weight loss. Goji berries may be the greatest source of antioxidants known.

In fruits and plant foods, sugars are combined with and balanced by other ingredients, such as structured water, vitamins, minerals, salts, and fiber, as well as other beneficial elements, known and unknown. It is not just a matter of a list of ingredients, but also the complex, life-giving structure of a whole food that makes the difference.

There are many natural, minimally processed sugars with most of their nutrients still intact, available at most health-food stores, to replace the white sugar you may have been using.

Raw Honey is the concentrated nectar of flowers that comes straight from the hive. An alkaline food, raw honey contains ingredients similar to those found in fruits, which become alkaline in the digestive tract. It has been collected by beekeepers since the dawn of civilization and is *EcoDiet's* number one recommended natural sweetener. Aristotle called it "the nectar of the gods." Just be sure to purchase it raw and organic. Most of the honey found in the supermarket is not raw honey but "commercial" regular honey, which has been pasteurized (heated at 70 degrees Celsius or more, followed by rapid cooling) and filtered so that it looks cleaner and smoother, more appealing on the shelf, and easier to handle and package. On the downside, when honey is heated, its delicate aromas, yeast and enzymes, which are responsible for activating vitamins and minerals, are partially destroyed.

Rapadura is a Portuguese name for dehydrated sugarcane juice. It is dried in the form of a brick and largely produced on site at sugarcane plantations in tropical regions. This process preserves all of the mineral-rich molasses, particularly silica.

Stevia is a low-calorie sweetener that comes in powder or liquid extract form. It comes from the leaves of several species of plants from the genus Stevia. It may be one of the best low-calorie sugar substitutes for the human body because it does not cause an insulin spike. Stevia has been shown to support the function of the pancreas, increasing enzyme availability and improving the body's ability to process other sugars.

However, beware of highly processed forms of stevia, processed chemicals extracted from the stevia plant, or products advertised as stevia but mixed with other sweeteners. They may have as little relation to the stevia leaf as white sugar has to a beet. For example, Rebiana (the tradename for rebaudioside A) is a chemical compound extracted from stevia through a 42-step process involving various solvents and patented by Cargill. Rebiana is one of the sweeteners found in Truvia®, touted as "a natural sweetener from the stevia leaf." There is nothing natural about Truvia®.

S-O-S QUESTIONS TO ASK YOURSELF

There are new sugars, salts, and oils springing up in the marketplace all the time. Before purchasing them, these are the questions to ask:

- Is this product a fresh whole-food or minimally processed?
- Is it certified organic?
- Does it come from a non-GMO source?
- Is a reputable company producing this product?
- If it carries a health-food company label, has it been acquired by one of the major food conglomerates such as Cargill, Coca-Cola, Kraft, or General Mills?

To avoid or reverse an ecological breakdown, heed your body's S-O-S signal and answer the call. That is, begin the process of alkalizing your internal environment by shifting to the right salts, oils, and sugars.

The next step is to eat as many alkalizing foods as possible every day. Then finally, feed your mind the strongest alkalizing thoughts you can think of and watch the shift into the *new you* take place!

Chapter 8

STOP ACIDIFYING AND START ALKALIZING

When you eat a diet high in fruits and vegetables, every cell of your body will be charged like an alkaline battery so that you, too, can keep going on and on and on and on...

Whether you're already experiencing an ecological breakdown caused by an acidic, low-oxygen environment, or simply want to prevent one, it's time to stop acidifying your body and start alkalizing. So now, let's delve into a more in-depth understanding of which foods acidify your internal environment and which foods alkalinize it.

STOP ACIDIFYING!

AN ACID ENVIRONMENT = A LOW OXYGENATED ENVIRONMENT

Sometimes the first thing required in changing deeply ingrained food habits is "just say no!" Most strongly acidifying foods are very addictive. Some people are addicted to cheese, others to Coca-Cola®. In order to truly nourish your body and restore your internal environment, you'll need to step out of the haze of addiction to strongly acidifying foods. When tempted, let "just say no" be your mantra.

STRONGLY ACIDIFYING FOODS AND DRINKS

All animal flesh and products; processed junk foods with
salt, oil, and sugar; condiments and nuts; chemical drinks.

Meat, eggs, and dairy—even if they are from organic, grass-fed, or cage-free animals—are strongly acid-ash forming foods and should always be avoided. (The exception is raw goat dairy, which is mildly alkaline.) These high-protein foods produce strong inorganic acids such as nitric, sulfuric, and phosphoric acid, which draw heavily on the body's alkaline reserves for neutralization before they are eliminated through the urine.

This is one of the many reasons why meat should be avoided. Over time, if too much animal protein is consumed without being replenished by alkaline, mineral electrolytes from whole plant foods, the body's alkaline reserves will be depleted.

For those of you who are not ready to shift to an all plant-based diet, just be sure to eat organic meat of free-range or pastured animals and organic, raw, dairy products from healthy, happy, pastured goats. In this way, you can at least try to avoid the added perils of bioaccumulation and biomagnification (the side effects of consuming toxic meat and milk from commercial, pesticide-laced feeds).

Highly refined, processed, or synthetic foods are metabolized differently. They leave little or no ash, but nevertheless have a strongly acidifying effect on the body. They force the body to metabolize glucose rapidly, which causes the cells to produce carbonic acid.

This is the same carbonic acid that ends up in the atmosphere from burning coal. We usually speak of carbon dioxide emissions, but excess carbon dioxide in the atmosphere combines with water molecules in the air, and in the tributaries and oceans, to form carbonic acid. In a general way, the same thing happens in our bodies, acidifying our tributaries.

In the human body, carbonic acid can be eliminated and exchanged with oxygen through the lungs and the breath, which explains why processed junk food does not draw down the alkaline mineral reserves of the body as strongly as animal flesh and products. So, if you must eat your mother-in-law's birthday cake, breathe!

Still, if you have any question about how rapidly and seriously your health can deteriorate from eating a diet high in junk foods, you might want to watch the documentary

Super-Size Me (Morgan Spurlock, 2004), in which Morgan documents his 30-day experience of eating only at McDonalds.

Mycotoxins. While mycotoxins aren't listed in the following charts, nor will you ever see mycotoxins (fumonisins, trichothecenes, or zearalenone, for example) listed as an ingredient on a box, they are ubiquitous poisons in our food supply. If you recall, mycotoxins are the highly carcinogenic chemical stress signals of various fungi. They are generally impervious to cooking or other types of food processing. Foods vulnerable to mycotoxin contamination include:

- grains and grain-based products, especially wheat, barley, oats, and rice
- corn (including popcorn), sugar beets and sugar cane, cottonseed
- flesh of grain-fed animals, especially pork
- milk and dairy products of grain-fed animals
- eggs
- apples, especially if the skin has been broken or damaged
- nuts, especially peanuts and pecans
- chocolate
- coffee
- beer and wine

Some of the ill effects or allergic reactions that people have to these foods may be due to a sensitivity to mold, more than to the food itself. Even if you don't have an obvious reaction, mycotoxins are highly acidifying and will damage your internal environment over time.

Here are a few tips for choosing coffee least likely to be contaminated by mycotoxins: avoid low-quality brands and blends, avoid decaf, choose Arabica beans, choose single estate coffee, choose organic, and look for manufacturers and packagers whose beans have been tested for mycotoxins, such as Dave Asprey's Upgraded™ Coffee.

Generally speaking, organically grown foods are a safer choice for minimizing your intake of pathogenic fungus and its chemical toxins.

STRONGLY ACIDIFYING FOODS LIST

Highly Refined Food Additives

Salt   Oil   Sugar   Artificial Sweeteners, Colors, Flavors, Preservatives

Highly Processed Junk Foods

Potato Chips	Theater Popcorn	Cheetos
Fried hamburgers	Fried Chicken	Fried Fish and Chips
French Fries	Nachos	Cheese Pizza
Breakfast Cereals	White Bread	White Rice
Semolina Pasta	Wheat Bread	Cookies
Cakes	Candy	Pies
Ice Cream	Pickles	Pickled Olives
Canned Foods	TV Dinners	Puddings

Processed Fruits

Canned Fruit w/Syrup	Jams	Jellies
Dried Fruits w/Sulfur		

Commercial Condiments

Distilled Vinegar	Ketchup	Mustard	Mayonnaise
Salad Dressings	Relish	Soy Sauce	
Bottled or Canned Sauces			

Note: While apple cider vinegar has an alkaline ash, distilled vinegar, an ingredient in most commercial condiments, is acidifying.

Nuts

Peanuts	Roasted Nuts	Pistachios	Cashews

Note: Peanuts and cashews (even the raw ones) are extremely acidic and should be eliminated from your diet. I have found that even a small handful of either of these can turn the next morning urine acid, no matter how many alkalizing foods I've consumed with them. Perhaps it is because peanuts and cashews are especially susceptible to contamination by aflatoxin, a common mycotoxin that is used to induce liver cancer in lab rats.

Fake Dairy

Cheese Dips	Processed Cheese	Margarine
Trans Fats of Every Kind		

Pasteurized Dairy Products

Milk	Cream Cheese	Yogurt	Cottage Cheese
Butter	Sour Cream		

Processed Meats

Sandwich Meats	Bologna	Spam	Hot Dogs
Ham	Bacon	Sausage	Smoked Meat
Pepperoni	Salami		

Domesticated Meat

Red Meat	Pork	Chicken	Bison	Veal
Organ Meats	Turkey	Lamb		

Wild Meat

Duck	Quail	Deer	Rabbit

Toxic Seafood

Top-of-the-food-chain fish and scavengers

Atlantic Cod	Atlantic Halibut, Flounder, Sole	Chilean Sea Bass
Cavier	Eel	Farmed or Atlantic Salmon
Shark	Imported King Crab	Orange Roughy
Atlantic Bluefin Tuna	Imported Farmed Shrimp	Imported "Catfish" (also called Basa, Swai or Tra)

Note: The Food and Water Watch created a dirty dozen list of the most toxic fish and seafood. This is the list shown in the table above. Keep up to date by getting the Smart Seafood Guide at http://documents.foodandwaterwatch.org.

STRONGLY ACIDIFYING DRINKS LIST

Drinks

Soft Drinks	Sports and Energy Drinks	Distilled Alcohol
Plastic Bottled Water	Fake Fruit Drinks	Powdered Drink Mixes

Soft Drinks

It is estimated that the average American drinks more than 53 gallons of carbonated soft drinks each year. This is more than any other beverage, including milk, beer, coffee, or water. Soft drinks are, unfortunately, among the most acidic and acidifying drinks we can consume. This is because:

- Carbon dioxide is added to make them fizz, and carbon dioxide added to water produces carbonic acid.

- In addition, many soft drinks contain phosphoric acid, which takes tremendous amounts of calcium to buffer.

- They contain either high amounts of sugar or high-fructose corn syrup, triggering the creation of additional carbonic acid, or toxic, acidifying sugar substitutes like aspartame, breakdown products of which include methanol and formaldehyde.

- Some contain BVO (brominated vegetable oil), which creates a cloudy, oily build-up in body tissues containing stored fat—and probably elsewhere.

- They may contain toxic chemical additives like the carcinogen 4-methyl-imidizole (4-MI) for caramel coloring and other synthetic coloring agents and preservatives.

- Many soft drinks contain caffeine, which is obtained as a byproduct of decaffeinated coffee. Caffeine is acidic, and draws down mineral reserves. It is addictive, depletes the adrenal glands, and causes long-term exhaustion.

- And finally, the aluminum can. Although most now have inner linings, the coatings are easily fractured. Soft drinks containing fluoride (from fluoridated water) will leach aluminum from the can.

The pH of these beverages varies with the amount of carbon dioxide and other ingredients in them, but it is generally extremely acidic, having a pH below 4. I have witnessed that it takes up to 35 glasses of strong ionized, alkaline water (pH 9.5), to neutralize the acid of just one cola or soft drink.

Product	Acid	Teaspoons of Sugar (in 12 oz.)
Sprite	3.42	9.0
Diet Coke	3.39	0.0
Mountain Dew	3.22	11.0
Gatorade	2.95	3.3
Hawaiian Fruit Punch	2.82	10.2
Coke Classic	2.63	9.3
Pepsi	2.49	9.8
BATTERY ACID	1.00	0.0

Laboratory tests, University of Minnesota School of Dentistry, 2000.
Arkansas Department of Health, Office of Oral Health, 2006.

Sports and Energy Drinks

Sports and so-called energy drinks are popular with some health-conscious folks. We have been sold on the idea that these drinks hydrate us better than water and are better for us than soft drinks. Unfortunately, especially where energy drinks are concerned, this is not true!

Drinking energy drinks during intense exercise can be dangerous. Energy drinks increase the likelihood of dehydration because caffeine is a diuretic and therefore causes fluid loss. At the same time, high sugar concentrations (above 8%) slow fluid absorption.

Popular sports drinks are formulated for rehydration, and may act as an initial quick fix for hydration, but according to Rob Faigin, author of *Natural Hormonal Enhancement*, "Most 'performance drinks' impair athletic performance, and most 'thirst quenchers' are actually designed to perpetuate thirst."

Let's look at the ingredients of a typical sports drink, Grape-flavored Gatorade®:

Water, sucrose syrup, glucose-fructose syrup (three forms of refined sugar for an immediate energy spike), citric acid (a diuretic that creates flavor and thirst), natural grape flavor with other natural flavors (MSG, maybe?), salt (refined, as a source of sodium), sodium citrate (another diuretic), monopotassium phosphate (a drug used to decrease the amount of ammonia in urine), synthetic coloring agents (red 40, blue 1).

It is a simple chemical stew with all that it implies: metabolic stress, acidification, and lowered oxygen levels. Besides the obvious, why is it likely to harm your performance?

- It contains more sodium than potassium. Potassium is essential for the conversion of sugars to glycogen, which is the fuel that powers each cell.
- Without adequate potassium, hydration of the cells cannot take place. Excess sodium promotes interstitial (between cells) water retention, which just acts as dead weight.
- It lacks other mineral electrolytes that are very important in athletic performance, such as magnesium, zinc, chromium, and selenium.
- The refined sugars promote spiking and dropping of blood sugar and insulin levels.

Not only do they fail to deliver true stamina, dental researchers are warning us that sports and energy drinks can be even worse than soft drinks in harming the teeth. Acidity causes most of the problems as acids alter the pH level in the mouth. When the pH level falls below 5.5, the bacteria that cause cavities proliferate.

In a study published in *General Dentistry* (2005), researchers soaked teeth in various popular drinks for a period of 14 hours. The drinks that caused the most enamel to dissolve included KMX® Energy Drink, Snapple® Lemonade, Red Bull®, Lemon-lime Gatorade®, PowerAde® Arctic Shatter, Arizona® Iced Tea, Fanta® Orange, and, finally, Pepsi® and Coca-Cola®. In fact, most popular soft drinks and sports drinks have a pH close to that of undiluted vinegar (pH 2.85).

The fake fruit drinks like SunnyD® (about 15% juice mixed with high fructose corn syrup, colorings and other chemicals) or Hawaiian Punch® (5% juice) are pumped up with huge amounts of sugar and more closely resemble a soda like Mountain Dew® than actual fruit. Don't be fooled!

"Plastic" Water

It's a fact; most bottled waters are acidic. I know because I've tested them all! Some companies have begun adding a pinch of mineral salts to their processed water to give it a better taste. But really, stop buying water off the shelf. If you need to carry water with you, buy an empty bottle (glass!) and fill it yourself with filtered, structured water from your home (more about this in *EcoDiet* Fuel Group #4, the water section of the *EcoDiet* program). I like the glass beverage bottles with a silicone sleeve that protects from breakage and provides a non-slip grip.

Popular bottled waters such as Penta®, Aquafina®, Dasani®, and Smartwater® have a pH of 4.0. Reverse osmosis or purified water from grocery-store machines may vary from 4.5 to 6.0. Not as bad as the energy, fake fruit, or soft drinks, but still! Why drink acid water? Even though some bottled waters may not have a strongly acid pH, drinking devitalized, chemically laced, "plastic water" will take you down the road to further acidification.

Bottled water sales are soaring, but in most cases, bottled water is no healthier than tap water. A four-year study by the Natural Resources Defense Council shows that one-third of the bottled water tested contains levels of contamination which exceed allowable city water limits.

Reverse Osmosis is a filtering process that is commonly used in bottled water facilities. The problem with this process is that some dangerous chemicals like pesticides, herbicides, and chlorine are molecularly smaller than water and can pass freely through the filter. At the same time, reverse osmosis removes healthy, naturally occurring minerals. These minerals not only provide good taste, they also serve a vital function in the body's system. When stripped of these minerals, water can become hungry, stripping minerals from the body in turn.

Then there's the bottle! Certain types of plastic leach dangerous chemicals, such as phthalates and bisphenol A. These chemicals seep into the bottled water, especially when the bottle is left in a hot car, a transportation truck, or left in storage crates out in the hot sun too long. Plastic toxins have been found to disrupt the endocrine system and cause fatigue, hormone imbalances, and weight gain. Both phthalates and bisphenol A, chemical components in some plastics, are endocrine disrupters for which a new term has been coined: *Obesogens.* You guessed it: water from plastic bottles can make you fat!

You can avoid a plastic toxin overdose by checking the resin code on the bottom of the bottle. This code tells you what type of plastic it is. Here is a quick rundown on the most commonly used and safest types of plastics.

PET (or PETE) 1: Polyethylene terephthalate has been deemed safe for one-time use, but refilling may increase risk of chemicals leaching out. Don't leave in the hot sun or re-use. A caveat: even if you are careful not to leave your bottled water in the hot sun, there is no guarantee that the manufacturer, shipper, or retailer hasn't left pallets of bottled water sitting in the sun or in a hot warehouse at some point.

HDPE 2: High-density polyethylene is commonly used for gallon jugs and has not been linked to any leaching.

PP5: Polypropylene is a plastic that is easily molded, meaning it is made with fewer chemicals than other plastics and has not been linked to leaching.

Plastics to avoid:

#3 Polyvinyl Chloride (PVC) has endocrine disruptors and probable human carcinogens. Its manufacture is linked to dioxins in the environment.

#6 Polystyrene (PS), as in Styrofoam cups, can leach styrene into food and water, especially when the contents are hot.

#7 Polycarbonate contains bisphenol A (a hormone disruptor). It is used in most baby bottles, five-gallon water jugs, and reusable sports bottles.

My advice: If you need to buy a bottle of water, look for a glass bottle!

MILDLY ACIDIFYING FOODS AND DRINKS

Organic grains, legumes, nuts, seeds, berries, and drinks

The foods in this section are what our great grandparents knew. They are heirloom varieties, organically or biodynamically grown. Conventionally grown foods don't really belong here because the chemical residues on or incorporated into the genetic structure of today's crops are in the category of strongly acidifying.

MILDLY ACIDIFYING FOODS AND DRINKS LIST

Organic Grains

Barley	Buckwheat	Kamut	Brown Rice	Wild Rice
Quinoa	Wheatberries	Oat Groats		

Organic Grain Products

Polenta	Popcorn	Corn Nuts	Oatmeal
Sprouted Bread	Rye Bread	Spelt Bread	Hemp Bread
Whole Grain Cracker	Whole Grain Pasta	Whole Grain Pancakes	

Note: Raw, gluten-free, or dehydrated crackers, and sprouted grain breads would be a more alkalizing and superior choice.

Organic Beans

Adzuki Beans	Black Beans	Black-eyed Peas	Lentils
Chickpeas	Fava Beans	Kidney Beans	Split Peas
Great Northern	Mung Beans	Navy Beans	Pinto Beans

Organic Soy Products

Soybeans	Edamame	Tofu	Soymilk and Yogurt

Note: While I'm not an advocate of soy products, they do not leave a strongly acid ash. Just be sure if you consume soy that you do so wisely, always avoiding GMO soy. Choose organic!

Organic Fermented Soy Products

Miso	Tempeh	Unpasteurized Soy Sauce

Organic Nuts

Acorn	Brazil	Chestnut	Filbert	Cashew
Hazelnut	Macadamia	Pecan	Walnut	

Organic Seeds

Poppy	Sesame	Sunflower	Pumpkin
Hemp	Chia	Flax	

Organic Fruits

Cranberries	Blueberries	Plums	Prunes
Raspberries	Blackberries		

Organic Vegetables

Corn	Winter Squash	White Asparagus Tips

Organic Condiments

Agar Agar	Ketchup	Mustard	Oil-free Salad Dressings
Horseradish	Pickles	Tapioca	Raw Apple Cider Vinegar

Organic, Raw Dairy Products

Cow Milk	Goat Cheese	Butter	Cow Cheese
Kefir	Yogurt	Cottage Cheese	

Note: While organic, raw dairy products tend to be only mildly acidic, I do not recommend them as a part of a transition to the EcoDiet food program.

Organic Drinks

Coffee	Beer	Wine

Grains and Legumes. If you're going to eat grains and beans, eat them in their whole form. Researchers have concluded that a relationship between whole grain intake and coronary heart disease is seen with a 20 to 40% reduction in risk for those who eat whole-grain foods habitually versus those who eat denatured, processed grains.

The key to making whole grains and beans more healthful is to soak them in water before sprouting or cooking. Grains don't need much soaking time—perhaps a few hours. Beans need a longer time, between 8 and 24 hours, depending on how fresh they are and the temperature in the kitchen. Soaking them in water neutralizes the phytotoxins in seeds, activates the digestive enzymes, and makes the nutrients, including fats, starches, complex sugars, and proteins, more available. Phytotoxins, that is, plant poisons, have a purpose. For example, phytates block seeds from sprouting prematurely, protease inhibitors act as natural insecticides, and they also inhibit the enzymes that help us digest protein. In sprouting seeds, including legumes, an amazing alchemical process takes place, which neutralizes phytotoxins and makes many more nutrients available, and there's no cost involved!

Note, however, that not all seeds will sprout under kitchen conditions. For detailed instructions on sprouting, see Ann Wigmore's definitive guide *The Sprouting Book* (Avery, 1986).

As you transition to the master phase of *EcoDiet*, remember that unsprouted grains and beans should ultimately be phased out.

Soy Products are questionable foods these days. While research is still being conducted on the health dangers versus the benefits of soy, there are clear indications that ingestion of soy isoflavones should never exceed 25 milligrams (the FDA's maximum safe amount) in any one day.

While I am personally not a fan of soy, I have concluded that the more healthful soy-food choices are fermented, predigested soy products like miso and tempeh that have been cultured for over a year. This is because during fermentation most of the highly toxic substances are broken down. Just make sure you are using soybean products that originate with organic soybeans since most of the North American soy crop is genetically modified (GMO) and treated with toxic chemicals.

Nuts and Seeds are fatty foods, which are typically the best sources of vitamin E, an immune-enhancing antioxidant and nerve protector. They also contain the largest quantity of fat of all unprocessed foods, much of it in the form of healthy polyunsaturated fat, so check for rancidity and eat them sparingly. Remember, polyunsaturated fat is the home of omega-3s and can be a highly nutritious component of fresh, whole foods. Many vitamins, minerals, amino acids, and carbohydrates round out the remarkable storehouses of nuts.

Paul Pitchford, author of the wonderful book *Healing with Whole Foods: Asian Traditions and Modern Nutrition*, says that "the seed is the spark of life, a living and perfect food." That spark is ignited, paradoxically, by water. Nuts are tree seeds also contain phytates, so they are best consumed after soaking for several hours.

Berries. Be aware that all acids are not the same. While there are certain acids, such as ellagic acid, in fruits like blueberries that make these fruits acid ash–forming, these superfoods were designed by nature to provide nutrients to inoculate and protect us. We take in these nutrients during their growing season (late summer, early fall) to protect us from certain flu strains and viruses that may appear in fall and winter.

A recent study found that a plant phytochemical found in blueberries strongly inhibited the replication of the influenza virus in cell cultures. Containing resveratrol, along with various polyphenols (antioxidants), berries are among nature's most powerful superfoods and are known to counteract heart disease, cancers, and other types of illnesses, in addition to viral infections. Plus, they are one of the few fruits that cannot be picked un-ripened, allowing it to accumulate its full spectrum of nutrients.

Cranberries, another acid-ash fruit, have been found to reduce the risk of heart disease. Studies have found that people who drink unsweetened cranberry juice have higher levels of good (HDL) cholesterol and improved blood-vessel function.

Nature prepares a table for us every season. Presented on that table are an array of fruits and their nutrient treasures, the potential of which has not been fully recognized or unleashed. We have lost the understanding of the power of nature's seasons and eating the fruits of those seasons. Those fruits sustain our energy and vitality during the season in which they ripen, but are also used in rebuilding our cells, strengthening our immune system against future challenges, and replenishing our internal storehouse.

The nature of some of the acid-ash berries, in particular, is that of inoculators against the kinds of bacterial and viral illnesses that appear in the seasons to come. Instead of running out and getting a flu shot, why not use nature's table as a preventative?

Coffee and Wine may have some healthful benefits in moderation. The pH of coffee tends to vary between 5.0 and 6.9. This variance depends on the blend of the coffee, where the beans come from, and if it was organically or conventionally grown. Soils from different regions have an effect on pH levels. This holds true with wine, as well. If you're going to drink wine, be sure to choose wisely to minimize added toxins. For example, choose wine produced by organic or biodynamic vineyards, without added sulfites.

ACIDIFYING THOUGHTS AND EMOTIONS

Oftentimes, it's not the type of foods you're eating that's causing an acidic pH, but what's eating you! Dr. Bruce Lipton, cell biologist and author of *The Biology of Belief*, has scientifically documented that strong negative thoughts and emotions greatly influence our biology. His research shows that genes and DNA do not control our biology, but that DNA is controlled by signals from outside the cell, including the energetic messages emanating from our positive and negative thoughts. Dr. Lipton's profoundly hopeful synthesis of the latest and best research in cell biology and quantum physics is being hailed as a major breakthrough showing that our bodies can be changed as we retrain our thinking.

He says, "Our genes are not programs that control our lives as taught in medical school; but are rather controlled by the organism's perception of our environment…When we change the way we respond to the environment we change our health and fate."

What I have found is that the illusion of separation (our disconnection from God, each other, and nature) and festering past hurts drive the insatiable urge to eat a diet high in acidifying foods—the stronger the emotional charge, the stronger the acid foods needed to numb ourselves. Toxic, acidic foods seem to keep traumatic patterning locked up in the body, like scum on top of a lake that holds toxicity intact, blocking the light.

Similar to eating acidifying foods over and over again, year after year, when you think and feel the same acidifying thoughts and emotions over and over again, year after year, your body continues to be adversely affected.

Eliminate acid thoughts and emotions from your diet and watch your biology change. After all, you are what you eat, and what you think and feel!

Acidifying Thoughts

I'm not enough	I'm confused	I hate my job
My spouse is not enough	Nobody loves me	I'm fat
What's the use	It's all my fault	Life is unfair
What's wrong with me	I'm worthless	I'm stupid

Acidifying Emotions

Resentment	Frustration	Jealousy	Hopelessness
Hatred	Insecurity	Anger	Loneliness
Unworthiness	Shame	Guilt	Fear

START ALKALIZING!

AN ALKALINE ENVIRONMENT = AN OXYGENATED ENVIRONMENT

This is where we move into the heart of an *EcoDiet*. If you're committed to improving the quality of fuel you feed your cells, the following lists of alkalizing foods are going to be very significant.

MILDLY ALKALIZING FOODS AND DRINKS

Mainly Fruits and vegetables

How many times have you been told to "eat your veggies"? And how about the adage, "An apple a day keeps the doctor away"? Scientific reports and studies are confirming that these sayings have a strong basis. Eating a diet high in fruits and vegetables is one of the best things you can do for your health.

Fresh, raw fruits and vegetables are bioelectrical in nature, as we are. They contain electrolytes and can actually be used to power small electrical devices. We need electrolytes for many reactions and transformations to take place in the body.

Fruits are also astringent, which means they have cleansing properties. If you want to keep your environment mopped up and sparkling clean, eat fruit!

Finally, most fruits and vegetables are alkalizing. Even strongly acid fruits like lemons leave an alkaline ash, which means they are highly beneficial to our bodies.

A study that measured the amount of various antioxidant chemicals in fruits and vegetables found that "the fruit extracts' antioxidant quality was better than the vitamin antioxidants and most pure phenols (another type of antioxidant), suggesting synergism among the antioxidants in the mixture." This means that you'll get more out of an apple than a vitamin pill!

Fruits and vegetables are not only alkalizing, they contain essential vitamins, minerals, fiber, and various other phytonutrients that keep you healthy. Compared with people who consume a diet with only small amounts of fruits and vegetables, those who eat generous amounts are likely to have reduced risk of chronic diseases, including stroke, cardiovascular diseases, and certain cancers.

Better yet, for those of you who have busy lives and believe that a fast-food drive-thru is your only grab-and-go option, you can change that perception right now. Fruits and vegetables are the ultimate fast food. With fruit, all you have to do is peel and go, and with vegetables all you have to do is wash and go. It's simple and deliciously alkalizing.

MILDLY ALKALIZING FOODS AND DRINKS LIST

Organic Fruits

Apples	Apricots	Avocados	Bananas	Cherries
Coconuts	Cantaloupe	Carob	Currants	Dates
Figs	Grapes	Grapefruit	Guavas	Kiwi
Kumquats	Lemons	Limes	Tamarind	Loquats
Mangoes	Melons	Nectarines	Olives	Oranges
Papayas	Passion Fruit	Peaches	Pears	Persimmons
Dried fruits	Pineapple	Pomegranates		

Organic Vegetables

Artichokes	Asparagus	Sprouted Seeds	Bamboo Shoots
Beets	Broccoli	Brussels Sprouts	Cabbages
Carrots	Celery	Cauliflower	Cucumber
Fennel	Eggplant	Garlic	Ginger
Green Beans	Horseradish	Leeks	Lettuce
Mushrooms	Okra	Onions	Parsley
Parsnips	Peas	Peppers	Potatoes
Pumpkin	Radishes	Rutabagas	Sea Vegetables
Sprouts	Squash	Sweet potatoes	Tomatoes
Turnips	Yams	Jerusalem Artichokes	

Organic Grains

Amaranth   Millet

Organic Beans

Lima beans   Navy beans

Organic Miscellaneous Items

Nutritional Yeast	Raw Cane Sugar	Raw Honey	Arrowroot
Kim Chi	Kudzu Root	Culinary Herbs	Raw Olives
Blackstrap Molasses	Sauerkraut	Umeboshi plums	
Almond Butter	Sun-dried Tomatoes	Most Spices	

Organic Nuts

Almonds   Chestnuts   Pine nuts

Organic Drinks

Red Wine   Almond Milk   Hempseed Milk   Coconut Milk
Herbal Teas   Fresh Juices and smoothies

Coconuts can be classified as a nut, seed, or fruit. To add to the mystery, even the "tree" that produces coconuts is not botanically classified as a tree. However, for the purposes of an *EcoDiet*, I would classify coconuts as one of the greatest of fruits. Like the avocado, it offers a high level and quality of fats and proteins. These two fruits could be called the "meat" of a semitropical *EcoDiet*.

I love the young Thai coconuts, but I recently learned that most of the conventionally grown Thai coconuts are:

- not fresh, but in transit by ship for up to two months;
- dipped in fungicides; and
- irradiated.

If you are fortunate enough to live in a place where you can have a coconut tree in your backyard or buy organic coconuts, then no worries. Otherwise, consider using frozen, organic, raw coconut water and coconut meat in your smoothies.

Raw Almonds are one of the few alkaline nuts. Therefore, while most nut butters are acidic to the body, raw almond butter is alkaline. Next time you're in the mood for a peanut-butter sandwich, try some raw, organic almond butter on organic sprouted bread instead. Peanuts are extremely acidifying while almonds are mildly alkalizing! And best of all, the kids love it!

But, there is the issue of actually finding raw almonds in the U.S. The USDA has mandated pasteurization of all almonds grown in the United States since 2007, even organic almonds. Some organic almond growers have gone to court to challenge this rule. Note that pasteurized almonds may still be labeled as raw. To find truly raw almonds, you'll have to look for imported brands.

STRONGLY ALKALIZING FOODS AND DRINKS
Leafy greens, green powders, and "green" drinks

Go Green with Dark-Green Leafy Vegetables! The strongly alkalizing foods are mostly green. Leafy greens are often the last vegetables we think of eating, but they are actually the first in nutrition. The leafy greens are a great way to boost your pH levels to new heights!

Dark-green leafy vegetables such as kale, Swiss chard, collard greens, spinach, dandelion greens, and more, provide a great variety of shades of green from the bluish-green of kale to the bright, kelly-green of spinach. Leafy greens run the whole gamut of flavors, from sweet to bitter, from peppery to tart.

The young, tender greens can be eaten directly out of the garden or in salads. The larger, more mature leaves can be chopped up, added to smoothies or juiced, and added to soups. Leafy greens provide a whole range of important nutrients and phytochemicals to keep us alkaline and healthy.

Greens contain a variety of powerful antioxidants that offer cancer-protective properties. In a Swedish study, it was reported that eating three or more servings a week of green leafy vegetables significantly reduced the risk of stomach cancer, the fourth most common cancer in the world. Greens have also been shown to significantly decrease the risk of breast cancer and skin cancer. These are just a few examples. In fact, drinking the juice of dark-green leafy plants is one of the quickest ways to alkalize the whole body.

One of the greatest features of leafy greens is that they contain high levels of chlorophyll. Chlorophyll is the green pigment in plants and algae responsible for capturing the light energy needed for photosynthesis. Green plants, like water, make life on planet Earth possible. When we drink the juice of chlorophyll-rich plants, it is like drinking liquid oxygen. The higher our oxygen levels the higher our vitality and the greater our immunity.

There's a mystery to ponder about our connection with green plants. Chlorophyll is identical to human blood with one exception: the element at the core of chlorophyll is magnesium, whereas the element at the core of hemoglobin (the main component of red blood cells) is iron. We think ourselves so different from plants, yet there are ways in which our make-up is remarkably similar.

In addition to folic acid, greens are known for a variety of powerful antioxidants that offer cancer-protective properties. They have also long been known as blood purifiers. Ann Wigmore describes how Dr. Yoshihide Hagiwara, a Japanese scientist who researched the healing power of green plants and grasses, reasoned that "since chlorophyll is soluble in fat particles, and since fat particles are absorbed directly into the blood via the lymphatic system, that chlorophyll can also be absorbed in this way. It is his opinion that once the chlorophyll molecule is absorbed, its magnesium ion is replaced with iron, making new hemoglobin."

Whether it is really such a simple replacement, or there is more to it, I believe that chlorophyll-rich foods are the perfect foods for the health of human blood. Leafy greens and green powders, such as barley and wheatgrass, are an important part of an ecotarian lifestyle.

STRONGLY ALKALIZING FOODS AND DRINKS LIST

Organic, Dark-Green Leafy Vegetables

Arugula	Beet Greens	Chicory	Collard	Dandelion
Endive	Escarole	Mustard	Kale	Parsley
Sorrel	Spinach	Swiss Chard	Watercress	

Organic Green Powders

Alfalfa	Barley Green	Wheatgrass	Kamut

Drinks

Alkaline water	Green Juices and Smoothies	Green Teas

ALKALIZING THOUGHTS AND EMOTIONS

Think about what an alkaline diet coupled with a diet of alkaline thoughts can do! Life-affirming thoughts and feelings have the power to alkalize your body just like fruits and leafy greens. Dr. M. Ted Morter, Jr., the great pioneer of acid-alkaline function and balance in the body, has this to say,

> Positive thoughts, memories, emotions, and beliefs can't overcome the negative effects of a constant acid-producing diet. And by the same token, a completely appropriate diet can't overcome the acid-producing effects of negative thoughts, memories, and emotions.

But together, think what they can do!

Dr. Mona Lisa Schulz is one of those rare people who can cross the borders of science, medicine, and mysticism. She is an MD, a practicing neuropsychiatrist, an associate professor of psychiatry at the University of Vermont School of Medicine, and a medical intuitive. She reports that people who have thought patterns such as, "I've got one health problem after another" notice physical changes in their bodies when they begin to affirm, "I love myself just the way I am." Instead of berating themselves for what they might consider to be problems and impediments in their health, they start loving themselves as they are and their bodies respond positively.

Think about it—don't we all respond better to love and acceptance than fear and criticism?

It has now been proven that just by thinking positive thoughts you actually create new neural pathways in your brain. When you start thinking positive thoughts about a situation you are facing, your body responds and begins to rewire the established negative patterns in your brain. Eventually, your brain starts operating from the new, positive alkalizing thoughts and translates them into physical reality.

Through her observations of MRI and PET scans, Dr. Schultz concluded:

Affirmations change the way our brains are wired and the brain lights up differently. So it's not just this flow, woo-woo stuff with purple, but it really has bio-chemical, neuro-chemical, neuropharmacological affects just as effective, if not more effective, than Prozac, Zoloft, whatever else you have.

If the thoughts that run through your head are mostly negative, your outlook on life is more than likely pessimistic; this type of attitude creates an acid pH and a desire for acid foods. Likewise, if your thoughts are mostly positive, you're likely an optimist; this type of attitude creates an alkaline pH and a desire for alkaline foods!

As you heal the traumas and beliefs of the past that drive your negative self-talk and gain greater psychological wholeness, you will have less need for acidifying foods that numb your feelings. You'll find that life is rich, and that natural, nourishing, living foods are deeply satisfying. The addictive cravings for highly processed salty, greasy, or sugary foods diminishes.

That's why I say, a plant-based, frugivore diet will not only transform the state of your physical health, but it will also transform the state of your mind and your emotions. It removes the veil and helps you remember who and what you really are!

My Motto:

When you feed your body the foods it was designed to eat, you are supporting your mind to have the positive, life-giving thoughts it was designed to think and the positive, life-giving emotions it was designed to feel. Change your diet and your thoughts and you'll change your life!

Whole foods = Whole thoughts = Whole emotions

So start by feeding your brain a diet high in the life-affirming foods and thoughts you were designed to "eat" and you will become the alkaline you that you were designed to be!

Alkalizing Thoughts

I AM enough

I seek to understand

There is always something to love about my work

I love my body as it is

My spouse is loveable as he/she is

I love everyone as best I can

I can do anything I put my heart to

I do my best to love myself the way I am

I AM worthy as I am

There are things in life that are good

I AM brilliant

I AM attaining my perfect weight by consuming healthy foods every day

Alkalizing Emotions

Happiness	Gratitude	Hope	Love
Peace	Inspiration	Self-Love	Joy
Worthiness	Compassion	Contentment	Humility

YOU ARE THE CHANGE!

Within the foods of the earth, and the "foods" of our thoughts and emotions, there are really just two sides of chemistry as Dr. Morse would say. One is the healing side of chemistry and the other is the corrosive (acid side) of chemistry. In restoring the ecological equilibrium of your internal environment, it's important to know how the things you take into yourself affect you—what moves you toward life and health and healing, and what moves you toward death and disease.

Having a sense of the acid-alkaline spectrum and where the foods you eat fall along that spectrum will provide you with a simple framework that can inform every choice you make. The pH spectrum is a major key.

There is another key to be found in the three simple ideas of S-O-S, and it's critical not to underestimate the power of these first steps. What might be interpreted as the baby steps of reforming your diet through attention to salt, oil, and sugar can actually be giant steps, and have huge implication your overall health and well-being. These steps will take you onto a new plateau from which you can launch the next stage of dietary evolution.

Salt, oil and sugar are "accessories" that we take for granted in our diet, and they easily become the fundamental framework that "flavors" everything. When you change the quality of your salt, oil, and sugar, you change the entire underlying framework of your diet, and suddenly you are in a new, expansive world of dietary possibility and health.

The conversation on dietary devolution may seem like just another litany of how bad things really are in our world, but it is meant to motivate you in new directions. After all, if you don't know what is making you ill, how can you change it? While the information itself will be useful to you in "navigating through the maze," I hope that it will also support you to question the foods that line the shelves of a grocery store—whether it is a conventional or health food store. If we are to move up the scale of dietary evolution, we must recognize the signs of deceit and corruption within our food supply—and also the signs that indicate a better world.

As hard as it is to sustain an unwavering gaze when looking at the dark shadows surrounding our agricultural practices, our food supply, and our medical system, it is important to make the effort to become aware. Even though it may be painful to consider, full awareness is the most powerful key you can imagine. Only when you are willing to really see what is happening in our world, both outer and inner, can you wield the true power of transformation.

Now that you have these three keys, I believe you are ready for the full unfolding of the *ecotarian* lifestyle. The dietary program that follows provides a four-fold framework—based on the ancient Greek perception of the elements—for natural feeding within the context of our modern lives. Though this program might seem unrecognizable to you, or our forebears, given what is necessary to create a resemblance of a "natural" lifestyle within our modern society, it is an attempt to return to our beginnings. For example, if we could still drink from pure bubbling brooks, we wouldn't need machines to purify our water. If we could pull our carrots straight out of the dirt or our tomatoes off of the vine from our non-toxic fields as I did as a child, we wouldn't need an organic seal.

The question I propose is this: Are you ready to become an internal environmentalist, an ecotarian—one who takes responsibility for the sustainability of their terrain and, therefore, that of the earth? Are you ready to take your place in the web of life on this earth? If so, read on.

PART THREE

THE ECODIET PROGRAM
How to Fuel Your Body for High Performance

Chapter 9

NATURE'S FOUR FUEL GROUPS

Start burning the right type of fuel into your internal environment and put an end to your environmental crisis!

Food isn't just something we put into our mouths and chew; it's any source of nutrients that fuels your cells. Food is dynamic, meaning that it interacts with its own forms as well as our body to produce energy. For long, food has been simplistically broken down into a food category classification known by most as the *Four Food Groups*, whose foundation is grains, fruits and vegetables, dairy, meat, and beans. This static representation of food fails to convey its essence and power. So, I propose relating to food in a nature's fuel approach. Rather than the Four Food Groups, I'd like to talk about the *Four Fuel Groups*, and they are rooted in the fundamental elements of earth, air, fire, and water. These four dynamic elements of nature are the very elements of our bodies, and they are the four groups that make up the *EcoDiet* Program.

EARTH, AIR, FIRE, WATER

Earth—the plant foods we eat from the earth comprise nature's first fuel group.

Air—the oxygen we breathe from the air is nature's second fuel group.

Fire—the light we absorb from the sun is nature's third fuel group.

Water—the water we drink is nature's fourth fuel group.

These four fuel groups were set in motion by nature from the beginning, each working together in perfect harmony with each other to keep the natural design of our internal environment alkaline, replete with oxygen, and completely alive.

Fuel your body with these dynamic four every day and either prevent or put an end to any internal environmental crisis you may be having. I did, and so can you!

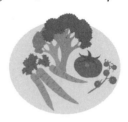

ECODIET FUEL GROUP #1—EARTH
FUEL YOUR BODY THROUGH THE POWER OF PLANT FOODS

Plant foods alkalize and oxygenize our internal environment like nothing else. This is because the healthiest, organic plants are grown in mineral-rich, pesticide-free soil with the support of sunlight, air, and water. Just as green plants saturate our planet's atmosphere with lots of oxygen, when we eat a diet high in alkaline, mineral-rich plant foods, they saturate our body's atmosphere with lots of oxygen.

With the *EcoDiet*, you'll be alkalizing your way to wellness because you'll be eating the foods you were originally designed to eat—foods that are alkaline to support our alkaline design. You'll also be following various other wellness principles that will assist your body in eliminating any accumulated toxic waste. Follow the Seven *EcoDiet* Principles for ninety days and you'll not only change the course of your life, but also the course of our planet!

THE SEVEN ECODIET PRINCIPLES

1. Eat a whole food, plant-based, alkaline diet.
2. Eat and drink raw, living foods.
3. Eat locally grown, seasonal foods.
4. Combine your foods properly.
5. Follow the circadian rhythm.
6. Feast and fast.
7. Follow the *EcoDiet* recipes for life.

EcoDiet Principle #1

Eat Whole, Plant Foods

The first *EcoDiet* Principle is to eat a whole foods, plant-based alkaline diet. This means that you will eliminate all processed foods, such as fast foods and pre-packaged foods (with a few minor exceptions), along with refined salt, sugar, and extracted oils from your diet. It also means that you will eliminate all animal foods, including eggs and dairy.

Instead, you will be eating all of the organic fruits and vegetables you can eat, with a small amount of nuts and seeds. These are the foods that come from seed-bearing plants and fruits. This makes you a true vegetarian, but better yet, it makes you an ecotarian, which means you are eating foods that support the sustainability of your internal environment.

No more store-bought dressings or sauces or meals in a bottle, box, or can. Instead, at the end of this section, you'll find a few simple and easy-to-follow whole-food recipes for oil-free, low-fat salad dressings, sauces, and meal ideas that I've created just for you!

Drink Whole-food, Plant-based Smoothies

Fruits, vegetables, and greens have abundant fiber—both soluble and insoluble. Fiber is good for cleaning the arteries and removing toxins from the body. Greens are a rich source of insoluble fiber. Green smoothies are a wonderful thing, but to make a smoothie with a creamy texture, add some fruits with soluble fiber. Bananas, pears, kiwis, strawberries, papayas, mangoes, avocados, and peaches are examples of fruits with soluble fiber.

Plants convert solar energy into complex chemical compounds called phytonutrients. Tens of thousands of these chemical compounds have been discovered. One of the best ways to be assured of getting phytonutrients such as flavonoids, bioflavonoids, or carotenoids, is to simply blend and drink it all—seeds, skin (with a few exceptions), and flesh! These nutritional powerhouses exhibit a cornucopia of health-giving benefits.

Eating a rainbow of fruits and vegetables every day also gives your body a wide range of valuable phytonutrients that science now knows will protect you from almost every chronic disease known.

Red Fruits and Vegetables are known for lycopene, quercetin, and other antioxidants that neutralize free radicals, regulate blood pressure, and reduce the risk of prostate cancer, among other things. Nature's red fruits include strawberries, cranberries, and watermelon. Red vegetables include red peppers, radishes, and beets.

Orange and Yellow Fruits and Vegetables contain beta-carotene, zeaxanthin, potassium, and vitamin C. They are abundant in antioxidants and other phytonutrients that are good for your skin, joints, eyes, and heart and also decrease your risk of cancer. Nature's orange and yellow fruits include oranges, mangoes, and peaches. Orange and yellow vegetables include sweet potatoes, corn, and pumpkin.

Blue and Purple Fruits and Vegetables contain lutein, resveratrol, and various flavonoids. Evidence indicates that these purple pigments protect our brains as we age, strengthen our immune system, support healthy digestion, and have anti-carcinogenic properties. Blue and purple fruits include blueberries, plums, and grapes. Blue and purple vegetables include eggplant, cabbage, and endive.

White Fruits and Vegetables contain allicin, an antifungal compound found in the garlic and onion family, and beta-glucans and lignans, which have powerful immune-boosting properties. These powerful phytochemicals are also known to balance hormones and reduce the risk of colon, breast, prostate, and hormone-related cancers. Nature's white fruits include bananas, pears, and dates. White vegetables include onions, potatoes, and cauliflower.

Green Fruits and Vegetables contain ample stores of chlorophyll, lutein, folate, and calcium. They neutralize free radicals, strengthen the immune system, regulate blood pressure, and reduce cancer risks. Does it sound familiar yet? Green fruits include avocados, kiwi, and honeydew melons. Green vegetables include leafy greens, asparagus, and peas.

These lists of the wondrous disease-fighting properties of phytonutrients are just the tip of the iceberg. Remember, in living foods, the whole is greater than the sum of the parts. Listing the properties of the known nutrients cannot give you the "whole" story. Get your medicine from blended, whole-food smoothies!

Drink Superfood Smoothies

Another group of phytonutrient-dense foods are called Superfoods. These are foods that have an extremely high phytonutrient content that may offer tremendous health benefits. These powerful superfoods are high in antioxidants and various nutrients proven to prevent and, in some cases, reverse the effects of aging and disease. Superfoods are so phytonutrient-dense that they also help to eliminate food cravings.

The following superfoods are possibly the most nutritious and powerful foods in the world.

Added to a morning smoothie, or made into a morning Superfood Shot, these foods will fuel your cell's engine for peak performance.

Green Powders are generally dehydrated green powders of young cereal grasses such as wheatgrass and barley grass. But, beware—not all green powders are the same. Some green powders are juiced before they're dehydrated, which gives you the highest form of nutrients possible. Other green powders are just freeze-dried whole plants, which leaves the fiber and destroys the enzymes. Green juice powders are the most nutrient dense, super-alkalizers, and blood purifiers known. The "superpowers" of green powders can be attributed, in part, to their high concentrations of chlorophyll, the liquid biofuel that oxygenates our body's atmosphere.

SevenPoint2™: The Alkaline Company makes a green powder blend that I recommend the most. The greens they use are not only of the highest quality possible, the taste of these greens far surpasses any powdered greens I've ever tasted. And best of all, your children will love them! The company's mission is the same as mine: to alkalize everyone on the planet, one bite at a time!

Superfood Berries are phytonutrient-rich berries such as goji, Acai, and camu camu. These berries are extremely high in dietary fiber, rich in fatty acids, and loaded with antioxidants. In addition, they contain healthy levels of monounsaturated fatty acid, oleic acid, omega-6, vitamin A, and calcium. Due to the highly perishable nature of the raw fruit, these berries, other than goji, may be available only in powder form. They make a wonderful super-charged addition to your morning smoothies. But choose raw (dehydrated at low temperatures), organic ones, and buy from a reputable company. Some manufacturers advertise the health-giving properties and list the nutrients of the fresh berry, but actually process them at high temperatures, destroying much of their nutritional value.

Nuts are powerful antioxidant and anti-inflammatory superfoods. Studies involving more than 220,000 people show that diets that include nuts help reduce the risk of heart disease, the leading killer of both men and women in the United States. As an example, the famous Seventh Day Adventists study followed the diets of more than 30,000 church members over a 12-year period. The results showed that, even in this healthy-living, largely vegetarian group, those who ate nuts at least five times per week cut their risk of dying from coronary heart disease by 48%, compared with those who ate nuts less than once weekly. They also cut their risk of a non-fatal heart attack by 51%. Always go for raw nuts, never roasted or salted, and don't overdo it. Nuts should still be a very small percentage of your diet, compared to fresh fruits and vegetables.

Seeds are among the phytonutrient-rich superfoods. Milk thistle, flax, chia, pumpkin, hemp, sunflower, and sesame seeds are high in fiber, vitamin E, and fatty acids. These health-promoting seeds are also great sources of protein, minerals, and other life-enhancing nutrients. Add a few seeds to your smoothie to provide a natural, whole-food source of oil.

Sprouts are among the top health-promoting superfoods. One of their many health benefits is the biochemistry that occurs during sprouting that transforms the seed into a plant, a process that unlocks the important resources stored in seeds that fuel a growing sprout. You can buy sprouts in the store, but commercial mung beans, for example, may be sprouted with chemicals and gasses in huge 500-gallon vats. The good news is that sprouting at home is fast and easy, so take a few minutes a day to sprout them in your own kitchen, under conditions that you can monitor yourself.

Maca Root Powder is considered by top researchers to be a true adaptogen (a natural herb product that is proposed to increase the body's ability to handle stress, trauma, anxiety, and fatigue). Each maca root contains more than 55 naturally occurring, beneficial phytochemicals. Working in tandem with the body's natural rhythms, maca root helps rebuild weak immune systems, balance hormones, re-mineralize poorly nourished bodies, and increase energy and endurance. Most people feel their mood and energy level lift in an instant.

Bee Pollen is one of nature's most powerful superfoods. Both the early Egyptian and early Chinese civilizations used it as a cure-all medicine for thousands of years. In fact, the Greek physician Hippocrates—widely recognized as the father of modern medicine—used bee pollen as a healing substance more than 2,500 years ago. Today, natural health-care practitioners often refer to bee pollen as a "fountain of youth;" it can be used for everything from weight loss to cancer prevention.

Royal Jelly is another superfood that has been revered as a "fountain of youth" since the dawn of history. The healing power and health benefits of royal jelly make it one of the most sought-after elixirs in modern times. It is hailed as the crown jewel of beehive products. A rich, creamy white opalescent liquid, royal jelly is produced by worker bees and used exclusively for the nourishment of the queen bee, who is recognized for her longevity (compared with regular worker bees: several years versus just 1 to 2 months), energy, and stamina for reproductive capability. Royal jelly is extremely high in nutritional value—especially natural hormones and amino acids, and is popular as a skin rejuvenator.

UMF Active Manuka Honey is considered to be an exceptionally healing honey. Collected from a plant that is unique to New Zealand, UMF Active Manuka honey is highly acclaimed for its medicinal properties. Manuka flowers appear in the spring and are much loved by the honeybees. Through scientifically based laboratory studies, this honey was found to have high levels of both peroxide activity (PA) from hydrogen peroxide which helps to oxygenate your body and non-peroxide antibacterial activity (NPA) which helps to rid your body of unfriendly bacteria. The letters UMF (Unique Manuka Factor) represent a standard of NPA antibacterial activity. While the active UMF component of Manuka honey is rated between 5+ and 25+, Manuka Honey USA has found that the best rating for internal use is 16+ to 19+.

Directions:

Green Powder
Take 1–2 tablespoons a day in fresh-squeezed juice or water.

Berry Powder
Take 2–3 tablespoons a day in your smoothie.

Nuts
Eat a small handful every day, except when juice fasting.

Seeds
Grind a variety into a powder and have a tablespoon a day in water or smoothie.

Sprouts
Add a handful to your salad every day.

Maca Root Powder
Take 1–2 tablespoons a day in juice or water.

Bee Pollen
Take 1–2 tablespoons a day right out of the jar!

Royal Jelly
Enjoy 1 tablespoon a day in a smoothie or right out of the jar!

UMF Active Manuka Honey +16
Enjoy 1–2 tablespoons a day in lemon water.

After drinking 16 to 32 ounces of purified water first thing in the morning, have a tablespoon of Royal Jelly, wait about 15 minutes, then try my organic Triple Superfood Shot. It is definitely a high-octane, alkalizing way to start the day!

Toni's Triple Superfood Shot

1 tablespoon green powder
¼ cup goji berries
1 tablespoon Acai berry powder
½ cup raw Noni or goji berry juice
1 tablespoon UMF Active Manuka honey +16
½ cup water

Place in blender and blend until smooth.
Note: Most of these ingredients can be found at your local health food store.

EcoDiet Principle #2

Eat Raw, Living Foods

The second *EcoDiet* Principle is to eat a diet high in raw, living foods. Eating a diet high in raw, living foods is the absolute healthiest way to eat. Raw, living foods include organic fruits, berries, wild and garden greens, vegetables of root and vine, sprouts, nuts, and seeds of every variety.

If 75 to 100% of your total food consumption consists of raw, living foods, you are considered a raw foodist, which is similar to an ecotarian. Both promote a lifestyle in which the majority of foods eaten are in their natural, whole-food, organic state—foods that are unprocessed and mostly uncooked. The greater the percentage of raw, living food in your diet the greater the health benefits.

Raw foods are considered "living" foods because they contain enzymes. Enzymes are a long string of amino acids that exist in every living thing that makes normal cellular function possible. They act as a catalyst for chemical reactions in cells, which simply means they either initiate or speed up these chemical processes. Many chemical processes require high speed to react properly, so you could look at enzymes as life supporting engines of cellular chemical reactions!

You and I depend on chemical reactions within the cells for proper function of the body and, in reality, for life. In fact, enzymes are the very things that make life possible. Without them, no hormone, vitamin, or mineral could do their work in the body.

This is where raw, living foods play a very significant role. When foods are consumed in their raw, living state, they contain high amounts of enzymes. Enzymes accelerate the flavor, color, texture, and nutritional changes in plant foods, especially when they are cut, sliced, crushed, bruised, and exposed to air. The process of an apple turning brown soon after being cut is a great example. Enzymes are also responsible for initiating the digestion of foods, which is the very reason that raw foods are so valuable to the body. They bring their own enzymes to the party, making it easier for our bodies to digest them, and to use the food's available nutrients. This is not the case for cooked foods.

Enzymes are very sensitive to heat above 118°F. When food is cooked, steamed, canned, pasteurized, baked, or boiled above 120°F, it loses virtually all of its enzyme activity. So, in the process of digestion, the body must borrow enzymes from the body rather than the food itself, resulting in a drain on our system. This is why you may feel sluggish after eating a cooked meal containing animal fat, and, by contrast, completely energized after consuming a raw green salad with fruit and nuts. The most nutritious way to consume your food is to blend it, juice it, or simply eat it raw!

Drink Raw, Living Juices

One of the fastest ways to restore your internal environment to a perfect state of health and well-being is to juice your way to wellness! Drinking freshly extracted green juices every day is like having a blood transfusion from nature's hospital. In fact, this is what I did 33 years ago to recover from my internal environmental crisis. After reading Dr. Norman Walker's book, *Fresh Vegetable and Fruit Juices*, I put my new juice machine to the test.

For 40 days, I drank 1 to 2 quarts of various vegetable and fruit juices along with plenty of pure water. After that, I continued drinking the same amount of juice, but I also ate a green leafy salad and some fresh, organic fruits in season. I ate no nuts, no seeds, no grains, no beans and, definitely, no extracted oils.

My family thought I had lost my mind, but what I had truly lost was an immune-deficient, disease-ridden body. The germ that had made my body its home had had its environment altered. With no food supply, it had no other choice but to pack up and go someplace else.

Fresh vegetable and fruit juices provide the body with an enormous amount of nutrients and phytonutrients for cleansing and rebuilding. It is the body's innate intelligence (sometimes referred to as the healer within) that knows how to restore ecological equilibrium when given the proper nutrients. I discovered that if you provide your body with the right materials in the right amount, it knows exactly how (because of this innate intelligence) to go about restoring health.

Here's a powerful juice your way to wellness tip:

> Citrus fruits are generally peeled, and many of us pick away at the white tissue surrounding the juicy segments to clean it all away. Turns out, though, that both the skin and the white tissue are especially rich in flavonoids—a phytonutrient that has great nutritional value. The parts that we generally throw away have been found to be anti-carcinogenic, anti-inflammatory, and have free-radical scavenging properties.

So put your juicer to work—put the whole fruit, peel and all, into your juicer and drink up! It's faster, easier, and definitely more highly nutritious!

So go ahead. Juice your way to wellness! I did, and so can you!

EcoDiet Principle #3
Eat Locally Grown, Seasonal Foods

The third *EcoDiet* Principle is to eat locally and seasonally. Food grown close to home is saturated with nutrition because it is picked close to its ripened peak. Eating locally and seasonally can be healthy for the environment as well. Buying foods purchased from your "food shed," loosely defined as farms within 100 miles of your home, helps to curtail global warming. Shipping and trucking food from all corners of the world uses millions of gallons of gasoline for transportation, and releases—not to mention—copious amounts of pollution into the environment, just getting to the supermarket.

Produce purchased from the supermarket has been in transit or cold-stored for days or weeks, whereas produce purchased from a local farmer's market has often been picked within 24 hours of your purchase. This freshness not only affects the flavor of your food, but the nutritional value as well, which declines with time and changes in temperature.

Spending your money at a local farmer's market is important for a multitude of reasons. It not only supports your health and the environment, but it also supports the livelihood of farmers in your community as well as the local economy.

Many farms offer produce subscriptions, where buyers receive a weekly or monthly basket of produce, flowers, fruits, eggs, milk, meats, or any sort of different farm products. Community Supported Agriculture (CSA) is a way for the food-buying public to create a relationship with a farm and to receive a weekly basket of produce. By making a financial commitment to a farm, people become members of the CSA.

Eat Seasonal Foods

A CSA season typically runs from late spring through early fall. Look at the body as having seasons, like the place where you live, and eat foods according to the ripening harvests of each season.

For example:

- *Autumn* is the time to eat lots of grapes, apples, persimmons, and other fall fruits, along with seasonal salads, steamed or roasted squashes, and other root vegetables.

- *Winter* is the time to focus on rest, meditation, and storing up energy. Strengthening, warming foods like soups and stews are good to eat (unless you live in the tropics).

- *Spring* is the time when a new cycle begins. A diet of more cleansing and revitalizing foods like dandelions, other leafy greens and sprouts harmonize the body in this season of rejuvenation and growth.

- *Summer* is the time when fruits are abundant, so a raw fruit diet low in fat is recommended.

What follows is a Seasonal Food Chart, with in-season fruits and vegetables listed for each season of the year. If you live in an area where your growing seasons are short, consider joining a company like Green Polka Box (listed in the Resource Section) that will ship seasonal organic produce grown in other parts of the country to your front door.

SEASONAL FOOD CHART

Spring (*March–May)*
Avocados, bananas, cherries, artichokes, asparagus, shallots, grapefruits, lemons, mangoes, broccoli, cabbage, cauliflower, navel oranges, papayas, pineapples, celery, cucumbers, garlic, apples, plums, strawberries, leeks, lettuce, mushrooms, raspberries, watercress, potatoes, rhubarb, snap beans, spinach, squash, onions, dandelion greens, parsnips, peas, herbs, carrots, beetroots, radishes, kale, watercress, parsley.

Summer (*June–August)*
Apricots, blueberries, artichokes, cabbage, carrots, peas, boysenberries, cantaloupes, zucchini, cauliflower, cherries, grapefruits, grapes, honeydew, celery, corn, cucumbers, lemons, nectarines, eggplant, garlic, peppers, peaches, Persian melons, strawberries, lettuce, mushrooms, okra, Valencia oranges, watermelons, onions, potatoes, spinach, gooseberries, mangoes, squash, tomatoes, watercress, radishes, raspberries.

Fall *(September–November)*

Apples, cantaloupes, dates, artichokes, broccoli, lettuce, cranberries, grapefruits, grapes, cabbage, carrots, celery, honeydews, lemons, plums, chili peppers, cucumbers, papayas, pears, blackberries, French beans, endive, leeks, Persian melons, persimmons, figs, escarole, peppers, peas, kale, kiwis, peaches, raspberries, parsnips, onions, yams, pumpkins, lettuce, potatoes, sweet potatoes, turnips, spinach, cauliflower, sweet corn, tomatoes, squash, watercress, chestnuts, beetroot, celeriac.

Winter *(December–February)*

Grapefruits, lemons, kiwis, navel oranges, artichokes, broccoli, cabbage, persimmons, tangelos, Brussels sprouts, cauliflower, tangerines, pears, celery, spinach, squash, turnips, lettuce, mushrooms, potatoes, tomatoes, parsnips, rutabaga.

Source: Compiled from the Third Street Farmer's Market in Santa Monica, California.

EcoDiet Principle #4

Proper Food Combining

The fourth *EcoDiet* Principle is to correctly combine the types of foods you eat. Some foods require different times and processes to digest than others, and thus should be eaten separately. Food-combining principles are as ancient as the dietary laws of the Mosaic Covenant; for instance, the Jewish law requiring the separation of meat and milk.

Fruits and non-starchy vegetables are digested quickly and easily. Other foods such as nuts and seeds require more time and specialized enzymatic functions. According to the studies of Dr. Herbert M. Shelton, the father of food combining and one of the greatest natural hygienists of the 21st century, there are sound physiological reasons for eating separately foods that require different digestive enzymes and gastric juices in the mouth, stomach, and small intestines.

The most important rule is to separate a meal of carbohydrate-rich foods such as bread, rice, cereals, and carrots from protein-rich foods such as beans, nuts, and animal products.

- Starchy foods require an alkaline digestive medium, which is supplied initially in the mouth by the enzyme ptyalin.

- Protein foods require an acid medium for digestion, which is supplied in the stomach by acid enzymes and hydrochloric acid.

Hydrochloric acid destroys ptyalin and suspends the digestion of starches. Undigested starch in the stomach interferes with the digestion of protein. It absorbs and neutralizes the enzyme pepsin, which is required for the digestion of protein.

In short, acid and alkaline digestive mediums neutralize each other. Therefore, if you eat a starch with a protein, digestion may be impaired or completely arrested, and undigested food can cause various kinds of digestive disorders. It becomes soil for unfriendly bacteria, which ferment and decompose, making poisonous by-products. One of these by-products is alcohol, which destroys or inhibits nerve function. Undigested food plays havoc with the nerves of the digestive tract, suspending their vital action; constipation may well be the end result.

Remember, also, to separate greasy and sugary foods. This means, don't eat fats with fruit or foods high in carbohydrates, such as grains or beans. An "oil spill" can clog cell membranes and inhibit insulin from escorting sugar into the cells for energy production. If you're going to eat a meal that contains extracted oils or animal fats, skip the dessert! Or skip the meal altogether! Or simply eat your fats such as olive oil, nuts, or avocadoes with greens or steamed veggies!

And finally, don't combine food with high stress! The nerves of the digestive system are highly sensitive to mental and emotional stress. Stress can paralyze digestive function.

As an ecotarian, you won't need to think much about food-combining laws or restrictions. When you are eating the way nature intended, proper food combining becomes a moot point. That is, if you were living out in nature, you'd be picking and eating whole fruit from the tree or the vine, and nibbling on some leafy greens. No problem!

It's as simple as that!

EcoDiet Principle #5
Follow the Circadian Rhythm

The fifth *EcoDiet* Principle is to follow certain daily cycles known as the circadian rhythm. Circadian refers to the regular recurrence of cycles of activity that occur approximately every 24 hours, or one full day. The rhythm is linked to the light-dark cycle. While sleep cycles are the most common studied by science, it has also been found that if one's daily eating patterns are in tune with these naturally occurring rhythms, people notice a tremendous increase in their overall health, energy, and well-being.

According to natural hygienists, there are three cycles associated with the circadian rhythm: (1) consumption (eating and digesting); (2) assimilation (extracting nutrients and assimilating); and (3) elimination (purging and releasing). Each has its own eight-hour period during which its activities are the most heightened.

> The *consumption* cycle is from noon until 8 pm. This is the time when the body is most capable of efficiently taking in and digesting food.

> The *assimilation* cycle is from 8 pm until 4 am. This is the time the body is extracting nutrients and assimilating what it needs.

> The *elimination* cycle is from 4 am until noon. This is the time when the body is gathering wastes and preparing them for elimination.

Step 1: The Consumption Cycle

Food should be eaten between noon and 8 pm. This is when your body is in the consumption cycle. The consumption cycle occurs when the body is predisposed to digesting food and allotting the energy to do so. In fact, Chinese medicine has long taught that our digestive fire increases and decreases according to the position of the sun. Thus, because the sun is at its greatest intensity from noon until 3 pm, these three hours are the most optimal time to consume the majority of our food.

Step 2: The Assimilation Cycle

Food should not be eaten between 8 pm and 4 am. This is when your body switches from the consumption cycle to the assimilation cycle and starts the process of extracting and assimilating the nutrients from the food you've eaten during the day. Hence, after the food you've consumed has been digested, energy is needed to extract and utilize the nutrients the body requires for optimal function. If food is eaten after 8 pm, your body is forced out of the assimilation cycle and back to the consumption cycle, diverting energy away from proper nutrient extraction and uptake and stressing your digestive system.

Step 3: The Elimination Cycle

Food other than fruit should not be eaten between 4 am to noon. This is when your body is in the elimination cycle. Food consumed prior to the completion of the elimination cycle not only severely retards the process of eliminating the accumulated wastes from the body; it also throws the rhythm of the three cycles into turmoil. The best way to flush out the accumulated waste during this cycle is to drink 16 to 32 ounces of purified water upon waking. Then eat only fruit until noon. Consuming fruit during this time does not disrupt the elimination cycle because the sugar component in fruit is a carbohydrate in its simplest form, glucose. It requires absolutely zero digestive energy to break down the sugar molecule and make use of the energy. Fruit also holds the plant kingdom's honor of being nature's greatest food for cleansing waste from the physical body.

EcoDiet Principle #6
Feasting and Fasting

The sixth *EcoDiet* Principle is to feast and fast. This is because the main function of blood cells is to distribute oxygen to every part of the body. But when we overeat, the blood is forced to act mainly as the body's feeding and waste removal system rather than a distribution center for oxygen. This means that instead of supplying the body with lots of oxygen, our blood cells must first get rid of excessive wastes from cellular oxidation. As we continue to overindulge, our bodies never have the opportunity to properly eliminate wastes, so our oxygen levels lower, our energy decreases, and disease sets in.

According to Ori Hofmekler, author of *The Warrior Diet,* recent studies have shown that both undereating (reducing calorie intake) and intermittent fasting have the potential to extend our life span and increase our resistance to almost every disease known.

Studying a range of organisms, from yeast and roundworms to rodents and monkeys, researchers showed that their maximum life span could be increased up to 50%, simply by underfeeding and intermittently fasting them. Researchers discovered that undereating reduced the incidence of neurological disease, age-related cancer, cardiovascular disease, and immune deficiencies in rodents while a high-calorie intake or overfeeding increased the risk for all degenerative diseases, such as cardiovascular disease, various types of cancers, Type 2 diabetes, and stroke.

Undereating was also shown to have a positive effect on brain function and debilitating diseases such as Alzheimer's, Parkinson's, and strokes. Undereating seems to protect neurons (a cell that transmits nerve impulses) against degeneration and stimulates the production of new neurons from stem cells, which may increase the ability of the brain to resist aging and restore function after an injury. While vitamins, minerals, and antioxidants may improve the health of the brain, it was shown that the major factor for brain health is undereating and an increase in the time between meals.

Researchers at the University of California, Berkeley, showed that healthy mice, given only 5% fewer calories than mice allowed to eat freely, experienced a significant reduction in cell proliferation in several tissues, considered an indicator for cancer risk. The key was that the mice eating 5% fewer calories were fed intermittently, or three days a week.

Cell proliferation is the increase in cellular division that takes place just before genetic repair is made, and cancer is essentially the uncontrolled division of cells. It was discovered that a cell will try to fix any damage that has occurred to its DNA, but if it divides before it has a chance to fix the damage, then that damage passes on to the offspring cells. Slowing down the rate of cell proliferation essentially buys time for the cells to repair genetic damage.

Substantial calorie reduction (up to 50% in some studies), not only reduces the rate of cell proliferation, but it can extend maximum life span from 30 up to 70% of a variety of organisms, including rats, flies, worms, and yeast. It was found that mice on a 33% reduced calorie diet exhibited significantly decreased cell proliferation rates for skin, breast, and T (lymphocyte) cells. The greatest effect was seen after one month on the regimen, when proliferation of skin cells registered only 61% of that for mice fed freely. The surprising finding came with the results of the more modest 5% reduced calorie diet that was fed intermittently. Mice in this group had skin cell division rates that were 81% of those for mice fed freely. So, even just a small reduction in calories makes a big difference in terms of your body's healing power.

Researchers discovered that fasting every other day also decreased the chance of breast cancer the most. In all cases, division rates for breast cells were reduced the most. Mice with the lowest calorie diet had breast cell proliferation results that were only 11% of those for the control group mice, and mice fed intermittently had results that were 37% of those for the control group. Undereating and intermittent fasting was also found to enhance insulin sensitivity and lower the risk of heart disease.

The problem? We're overtaxing our digestive systems. The body needs time to digest, assimilate, and eliminate waste. If waste is allowed to accumulate, our internal waters become toxic and acidic.

The solution? Eat less and fast often on organic vegetable and fruit juices, giving your digestive system time to fully process what you bring in and have to eliminate. This gives your body time for some much needed "house cleaning!" When your internal environment is "swept free" of waste, your body will be functioning at peak performance.

The following is the feasting and fasting protocol I like to adhere to the majority of the time:

Eat during a 4-hour daily cycle only. Drink your favorite freshly-prepared juice or lemon water until 12 pm. Then eat meals of solid foods only between 12 pm and 4 pm. If you feel hungry after 4 pm, enjoy more freshly-prepared juice. This will give your body a 20-hour fast every day. If you follow this simple guideline, you'll be amazed at how great you feel!

BUT WHAT IF I'M HUNGRY?
Eat Light!

When you begin to feast and fast, it is normal to feel a little hungry between meals. Over the years, our bodies have adapted to eating three "square" meals a day! However, if you feel constantly hungry and tend to gain weight in the wintertime, try a little sunlight! Melatonin, triggered by darkness, can cause an increase in appetite. Low levels of vitamin D from lack of sunlight can trigger fat storage. Brave the cold and get outside for 15 to 20 minutes a day. Go out when the sun is highest in the sky. Try wearing a down vest while leaving your forearms exposed to the light.

So, eat light! You'll be glad you did!

EcoDiet Principle #7
Eat Your Way to Wellness

The seventh *EcoDiet* Principle is to show you what it means to burn the right type of food for fuel. Just as the grade of gasoline we burn in our car's engine affects the outer environment in a positive or negative way, the grade of food we burn in our body's engine affects our internal environment in a positive or negative way. Gasoline is classified by three grades: regular, midgrade, and premium. Likewise, food fuel can be classified by these same three grades, which are explained below.

Before we move forward, however, let me emphasize that the most important thing in terms of health is to just get started; choose one of the levels, regardless of what you are currently prepared to "give up" (or not) at this stage. All the levels are vegetarian and all are free from processed foods, therefore, offering far better nutritional support for the human body than non-vegetarian diets. But it is not essential—unless you are suffering from a serious health disorder—for you to follow these diets precisely in order to benefit.

For example, if you choose to eat meat a couple of times a week, then make sure it's organically-raised and do it within the structure of one of the levels below, and you will realize great benefits. Similarly, if you function well in Level Two and realize that you benefit from eating eggs or beans every once in a while, then be okay with that. As I said previously, taking time to incorporate dietary changes can be very beneficial; I have found that change becomes more permanent when practiced over time. Obviously, strict adherence to the parameters outlined below will provide the greatest benefits, and are important if you are ill, but you don't have to be perfect to win! And…remember to go easy on yourself; positive thoughts are a key alkalizing factor, and essential for good health. So, let's get started!

> *Regular is classified as Level One.* This diet is the Beginner Vegetarian Plan, for the person transitioning from an omnivorous diet.
>
> *Midgrade is classified as Level Two.* This diet is the Intermediate to Advanced Vegan Plan.
>
> *Premium is classified as Level Three.* This diet is the Master Ecotarian Plan.

LEVEL ONE
The Beginner Vegetarian Plan

> 80% Alkaline Foods/20% Mildly Acid Foods
> 50% Raw/50% Cooked

Level One is regular fuel—the beginner vegetarian fare. It's a transitional diet for those who have been eating a highly acidic, animal-based, processed-food diet. This plan is a plant-based, organic, whole-foods diet that places emphasis on fruits and vegetables, gluten-free grains, beans, nuts, seeds, and a small amount of raw goat dairy. It is animal-free, gluten-free, processed food-free. On this plan, you would follow the 80/20 Plan—80% alkalizing foods and 20% mildly acidifying foods; 50% raw and 50% cooked. (Note: If you test positive for candida, go directly to Level Three, the premium fuel.)

This means:

1. No processed foods (with a few exceptions).
2. No animal meats.
3. A few organic, free-range eggs from time to time.
4. No cow dairy products, but raw goat dairy is acceptable but limited.
5. Eat all the fruits and vegetables you desire.
6. Include a small amount of gluten-free grains, beans, nuts, and seeds.
7. Include a small amount of Celtic sea salt, olive and coconut oils, and natural sweeteners like honey.

Follow the seasons of change:

- Eat a mostly raw-food diet in the spring and summer, enjoying lots of seasonal fruits, greens, and vegetables along with a small amount of nuts and seeds. Always keep your fat intake in the spring and summertime extremely low.

- Eat more cooked foods in the autumn and winter (unless you live in the tropics!), adding in steamed, roasted, or grilled seasonal vegetables, and a small amount of raw goat dairy, gluten-free grains, beans, nuts, and seeds.

Follow the circadian rhythm:

- Fruits are powerful breakfast foods for cleaning out acidic waste during the elimination cycle.

- Vegetables are the most powerful lunch and dinner foods for alkalizing your body during the consumption cycle.

Feast and fast:

- Take one day a week to fast on freshly-prepared juices only. Choose any of your favorites listed in the recipe section that follows.

To be more specific, your Level One daily menu would look like this:

- For breakfast, you might enjoy a large bowl of fruits or a smoothie, using fruits grown in season.

- For lunch or dinner, enjoy a large plate of leafy green salad, steamed or roasted veggies, and a small portion of beans, brown rice or brown rice pasta.

Imagine looking at your lunch or dinner plate. At least 80% of the foods you see on your plate are foods from the alkaline food lists and up to 20% could be foods from the mildly acidifying food lists: 50% of your daily plan would be eaten fresh and raw; 50% would be eaten lightly grilled, baked, or steamed.

Level One—Sample Menu Ideas

BREAKFAST IDEAS

The first meal of the day is a fruitarian fare. Enjoy a bowl of seasonal fruits, a smoothie, or freshly-prepared juice. Remember that fruits are cleansing and are great foods to consume during the morning elimination cycle. So enjoy as much as you want!

- Blend up a fruit smoothie with 2 cups of raw coconut water and any fruit in season. One of my favorites is very simple: fresh pineapple and raw coconut water.

- How about a delicious fruit salad with your favorite fruits in season? Enjoy it plain or drizzle with date sauce (4 Medjool dates, 1 cup water, and blend until creamy).

- Try blending 1 banana and several pitted dates with a cup of water; if it is wintertime and you want to warm yourself up, try adding a few shakes of cayenne pepper!

- Have a *Green Smoothie*. Blend a handful of stemmed kale or spinach with your choice of fresh organic, soluble-fiber fruit, such as mango, banana, or pear, and water. The soluble fiber makes for a creamy textured smoothie.

- Or, if you're like most and don't have a lot of time in the morning, simply add 1 to 2 tablespoons of my favorite *SevenPoint2* Greens to your smoothie recipe of choice! You'll be glad you did!

- Why not begin your day with one of my favorite juices? Juice 2 apples, 1 unpeeled lemon, a 1-inch piece of fresh ginger, 2 ounces wheatgrass juice; then, if you want to take it up a "hot notch," add ½ habanera pepper.

- Sometimes, I just like to keep it simple: one fruit at a time. Try a bowl of mangoes or papayas, grapes, peaches, pears, or some watermelon, whichever fruit is in season.

- Or, simply juice 1 whole lemon (peel and all), add it to a quart jar with 2 tablespoons Active Manuka Honey, fill with water, shake and drink. This will start your day cleaning out the accumulated acid wastes!

LUNCH IDEAS

The main meal of the day is a heavier vegetarian fare with lots of vegetables and a small amount of rice, beans, or gluten-free pasta. Enjoy all of the alkalizing vegetables you want!

- My favorite transitional meal is a small amount of gluten-free brown rice pasta tossed with a small amount of olive oil, crushed garlic, and salt. Add some freshly chopped basil and lots of cherry tomatoes cut in quarters. Toss again, then serve over a large bed of baby arugula.

- For a delicious Italian taste-bud delight, create a bountiful bowl of organic Roma tomatoes cut in quarters, tossed with Cannellini beans, salt, raw goat cheese, roasted red peppers, and garlic; all stacked high on a plate of chopped radicchio and frisse leaves.

- For a Greek delight, create a bowl of Fava beans, thinly sliced red onion, chopped up basil leaves, several handfuls of baby arugula, raw goat cheese, salt, and olive oil.

- Or, how about a Greek salad with sliced cucumbers, green bell peppers, tomatoes, red onion slivers, raw goat feta, a dash of dill, oregano, salt, and olive oil with a large serving of roasted veggies?

- If it's wintertime, enjoy a bowl of red beans, cayenne pepper, and escarole greens, tossed with lots of chopped avocado.

- How about a large bowl full of heirloom black rice, grilled asparagus, over a bed of finely chopped radicchio, tossed in your favorite oil-free dressing?

DINNER IDEAS

The last meal of the day is a lighter vegetarian fare: soup, salad, or both. Most of these ideas can be found in the recipe section that follows. If not, use your imagination—create your own!

- Have a large leafy green salad tossed with steamed potato cubes, avocado, grape tomatoes, pressed garlic, salt, and olive oil.

- If you're a potato lover, enjoy a bowl of *Potato Corn Soup* served with *Over The Rainbow Salad*.

- How about a large arugula salad tossed with slices of sun-dried tomatoes, chopped raw olives, organic capers, raw goat feta, tossed in olive oil, along with a bowl of *Roasted Red Bell Pepper Bean Soup*?

- For an Italian Feast, try an *Italian Potato Salad* featuring fingerling potatoes, sliced red bell peppers, tossed in pressed garlic, salt, and olive oil, and roasted in the oven until potatoes are slightly brown; then tossed with arugula. Delicious!

- For a Mexican feast, enjoy a large *Salsa Wrap* (salsa wrapped in a large lettuce leaf) tonight with a bowl of *Black Bean Soup*.

- If it's cold outside and you want something to warm your bones, how about a bowl of *Vegetable Bean Chili* with your salad of choice?

- If it's springtime, enjoy a large *Butter-Me-Up Salad* with a bowl of *Asparagus Miso Soup*.

LEVEL TWO
The Intermediate to Advanced Vegan Plan

Low-Fat, Oil-Free
80% Alkaline Foods/20% Mildly Acid Foods

Intermediate
50% Raw/50% Cooked

Advanced
80% Raw/20% Cooked

Level Two is midgrade fuel—the intermediate and more advanced vegan fare. It is a diet for those who have been following the Level One plan for several months and are ready to take that next step, or for those who aren't (or haven't been) fond of consuming animal products and want to jump right in! This plan consists of a plant-based, organic, whole-foods diet that places emphasis on equal proportions of fruits and vegetables, and a small amount of nuts and seeds. This diet is animal-free, dairy-free, oil-free, processed-food free, grain-free, and bean-free. On this plan, 80% of your foods will be from the alkaline food list and 20% mildly acid foods in the form of nuts and seeds only—and either: 50% raw and 50% cooked, or 80% raw and 20% cooked. Obviously, the more raw foods the better for the *EcoDiet*!

*The main difference between Level One and Level Two
is that you'll be eliminating raw goat dairy,
extracted oils, grains, and beans.*

This means:

1. No processed foods (with a few exceptions).
2. No animal meats.
3. No eggs.
4. No dairy products, including no dairy from goats.
5. No grains or beans.
6. No extracted oils.

7. Eat all the fruits and vegetables you desire, including root vegetables.

8. Include a small amount of nuts, seeds, and olive and coconut oil.

Follow the seasons of change:

- Eat a mostly raw food diet in the spring and summer, enjoying lots of seasonal fruits and vegetables, along with a small amount of nuts and seeds.

- Eat a few more cooked foods in the autumn and winter (unless you live in the tropics!), adding in more steamed, roasted, or grilled seasonal vegetables, including root vegetables, and a small amount of nuts, seeds, and salt.

Follow the circadian rhythm:

- Fruits are powerful breakfast foods for cleaning out acidic waste during the elimination cycle.

- Vegetables, especially leafy greens, are the most powerful lunch and dinner foods for alkalizing your body during the consumption cycle.

Feast and fast:

- Take one day a week to fast on freshly-prepared juices or water only. Choose any of your favorites listed in the recipe section that follows.

To be more specific, your Level Two daily menu would look like this:

- For breakfast, juice until 12 pm, or simply eat fruit or enjoy a smoothie.

- For lunch or dinner, you might enjoy a large leafy green salad, your favorite oil-free dressing, topped with steamed or roasted veggies.

Imagine looking at a plate of food. Simply put, at least 80% of the foods you see on your plate would be fruits and veggies from the alkaline food lists and 20% would be foods from the mildly acid food list in the form of nuts and seeds only: 80% of your daily fare would be eaten fresh and raw; 20% would be eaten lightly grilled, baked, or steamed—or 50/50 if you're on the intermediate plan. For example, the food on your lunch plate would consist of a large green leafy salad with a baked russet or sweet potato, raw or lightly steamed vegetables on the side.

Level Two—Sample Menu Ideas

BREAKFAST IDEAS

For a fruitarian fare, start your day with your favorite seasonal fruits. Go ahead! Eat them, blend them, or juice them. You can use the same breakfast ideas from Level One for your Level Two. Need a few more ideas? Try these!

- Try one of my *Superfood Fruit Smoothies*, or use your own creative imagination. How about creating your smoothie with 2 to 3 different fruits such as a whole apple, banana, and orange along with 2 to 3 cups of water. Go ahead; blend the whole fruit, skin, seeds and all; the skins and seeds are loaded with phytonutrients. Add your favorite superfood raw, dehydrated juice powders such as Acai or goji berries, or raw green powder blend.

- I love berries, and they are loaded with antioxidants, so how about a *Berry Good Blend*? Blend ½ cup of fresh organic raspberries, blueberries, strawberries, and blackberries with 2–3 cups of water; add a frozen banana and a superfood powder or juice blend. Go ahead; get creative!

- Take yourself to the tropics one morning with a *Tropical Treat*—blend 1 cup fresh organic pineapple, mango, and papaya with lots of fresh young coconut water and coconut meat. Add a banana and blend!

- Have a *Lean-Green Smoothie*—for a highly concentrated dose of chlorophyll, blend a handful of stemmed dinosaur kale, 1 to 2 tablespoons of *SevenPoint2* Greens with your choice of soluble-fiber fruit, such as mango or banana, and 3 cups purified water or raw coconut water.

LUNCH IDEAS

This meal is designed to be the heaviest vegan fare of the day. Enjoy all of the vegetables your heart desires! Vegetables are alkalizing and are the majority of foods to consume during the second food cycle of the day: the consumption cycle. So enjoy as much as you want. Feel free to always add a few raw nuts or sprouted seeds on top! For those of you on the intermediate or advanced vegan program, simply factor in your cooked to raw ratio.

- How about a living lentil salad? Place a cup of sprouted lentils tossed with pressed garlic, salt, avocados, grape tomatoes, red onion slivers onto your plate and eat your way to garlic heaven. Enjoy a small amount of steamed veggies.

- How about a large bowl of your favorite leafy greens, topped with steamed or roasted organic fingerling potatoes tossed with pressed garlic, and salt?

- For a simple yet delicious meal in a bowl, create a bountiful bowl of your favorite chopped veggies, red fingerling potatoes tossed with a dash of salt, chopped parsley, mint, dill, green onions, avocado, and tomatoes.

- Try a large bowl of leafy greens topped with your favorite raw and steamed veggies and a drizzle of sweet oil-free dressing?

- For a delicious Italian delight, create a bountiful bowl of organic Roma tomatoes cut in quarters, tossed with roasted red peppers, chopped basil, salt, garlic, stacked high on a plate of chopped radicchio and frisse leaves— drizzled with your favorite oil-free dressing.

- For an autumn feast, how about a baked yam drizzled in raw honey, with a large raw veggie chop salad on the side?

- Or, how about a raw vegan Greek salad with sliced cucumbers, green bell peppers, tomatoes, red onion slivers, a dash of dill, oregano, salt, and a side of roasted veggies?

- If it's springtime, you might enjoy a large asparagus salad featuring lots of steamed or raw asparagus pieces, sliced cherry tomatoes, diced Valencia oranges, chopped shallots, all tossed in your favorite oil-free dressing, or simply tossed in lemon juice and tarragon.

DINNER IDEAS

The last meal of the day is a lighter vegan fare featuring soup and salad. Most of these ideas can be found in the recipe section that follows. If not, use your imagination…create your own! Again, for those of you on the intermediate or advanced vegan program, simply factor in your cooked to raw ratio.

- If you're a tomato lover like me, enjoy a bowl of *Tomato-Basil Soup* served with any of the salads found in the recipe section of this book.

- If it's summertime, enjoy a small bowl of *Vegetable Soup* served with a large chopped veggie salad.

- How about a large mixed green salad with lots of avocado and tomato, all tossed in your favorite oil-free dressing and a small bowl of *Cream of Broccoli*?

- If you're feeling like creating balance in your life, try a large *Yin Yang Salad* with a small bowl of *Coconut Curry Soup*. You'll be glad you did!

- If it's springtime, enjoy a large *Watercress Papaya Salad* with a bowl of your favorite soup.

- Or simply enjoy a bowl of "energy soup" made with a handful of baby greens, 1–2 cups of sunflower sprouts, ½ avocado, 1 whole apple (peel, seeds and all), and raw coconut water.

- If it's wintertime, enjoy a large chopped veggie salad with a hot bowl of *Fennel Potato Soup*.

LEVEL THREE
The Master Ecotarian Plan

Low-Fat, Oil-Free
95% Alkaline Foods/5% Mildly Acid Foods
100% Raw

Level Three is premium fuel—the master ecotarian fare. It consists of a plant-based, organic, whole and raw food diet that places emphasis on fruits, dark leafy greens, non-starch vegetables, and a small amount of nuts and seeds. This diet is animal-free, dairy-free, grain-free, bean-free, starch-free, salt-free, and oil-free. Over time, this plan will clean the accumulated acids out of your body and alkalize you quickly. It's for those of you who are ready to go for the highest state of health possible. Try it, even if it's just for 90 days, and see what I mean!

On this plan, you would follow the 95/5 Plan, but this time it looks like this: 95% alkaline foods in the form of fruits and vegetables, and 5% mildly acid foods in the form of nuts and seeds—100% raw.

The main difference between Level Two and Level Three is that you'll be increasing your intake of fruits and vegetables, eliminating potatoes and salt, and eating everything raw.

This means:

1. No processed foods (with a few whole food exceptions).
2. No animal meats.
3. No dairy or eggs.
4. No grains or beans.
5. No potatoes or other starchy vegetables such as winter squashes.
6. No salt or oil.
7. Eat all the fruits and vegetables you desire.
8. Include a small amount of nuts and seeds.

Follow the seasons of change:

- Eat a mostly raw fruit and vegetable (including greens) diet during all four seasons, for breakfast and lunch, with a large leafy green, vegetable salad for dinner.

- Always keep in mind to vary your foods from season to season. And again, unless you live in the Bahamas, Florida, or southern California, if it's summertime, you'll naturally want to eat a lot of fruit and less fat than you would in the wintertime. In springtime, focus more on spring greens like watercress, dandelion, and sprouts; after all, everything is turning green and sprouting in the spring. In the wintertime, eat a little less astringent fruit and more fatty fruits like avocado and coconut, and a few more vegetables than you would in the summertime. Just remember to shift your food choices with each season of change.

Follow the circadian rhythm:

- Fruits are powerful breakfast foods for cleaning out acidic waste during the elimination cycle but can also be enjoyed during lunch.

- Enjoy lots of green leafy salads for dinner during the consumption cycle.

Feast and fast:

- Take one day a week to fast on water or freshly-prepared juices or water only. Choose any of your favorites listed in the recipe section that follows.

To be more specific, your Level One daily menu would look like this:

- For breakfast, enjoy a quart (32 ounces) of freshly-prepared juice or fruit salad.

- For lunch, enjoy a bowl of seasonal fruits, green smoothie, or a large veggie salad with your favorite oil-free dressing.

- For dinner, enjoy a large bowl of raw soup with a leafy green vegetable salad.

Imagine looking at your lunch or dinner plate. Simply put, the foods you see on your plate would be fruits, leafy greens, and/or vegetables, all tossed with an oil-free salad dressing—100% of your daily fare would be eaten fresh and raw.

And no! You don't have to spend hours in the kitchen prepping, dehydrating, and preparing fancy raw-food meals; that is, unless you want to. All you have to do is pick, peel, and eat—just as if you were living out in nature. Or, if you want some raw food chips with your raw soup, try *Brad's Raw Chips* that are already premade for you and found at most health food stores!

Simply keep in mind that the reason you eat is to fuel the trillions of cells that swim throughout the waters of your body with foods that supply them with lots of energizing fuel. Fruits, greens, vegetables, along with a small amount of nuts and seeds, are the premium fuel foods!

To show you how really simple it is, here's a sample week of menu ideas:

Level Three—Sample Menu Ideas
BREAKFAST IDEAS

Seasonal fruits are the main fuel for breakfast. It's the time of the day your body needs to not only eliminate any toxic, accumulated waste, but it's also the time every cell in your body requires the extra high-octane energy that only fruits can give.

- Enjoy as much freshly prepared juice as you want for breakfast.

- If it's summertime, eat as much watermelon as you want!

- Have a *Banana Date Smoothie*: Blend 2 bananas with 3 Medjool dates in 16 ounces of water. Simply delicious!

- What about a *Tropical Delight?* Blend 1 large mango, 1 banana, 1 small papaya with 1-2 cups of raw coconut water.

- How about a *Berry Good Smoothie* today? Blend 1 banana, 1 cup blueberries, 1 cup strawberries, 1 cup raspberries with the juice of 3 oranges.

- Try a *Mango Mania Smoothie* today: Blend 3 mangoes, 1 banana, with 16 ounces of coconut water and enjoy.

- At least once a week, I enjoy a very simple *Pineapple Coconut Smoothie* for breakfast: I simply blend 1 quart pineapple pieces with 20 ounces raw coconut water.

- How about a simple blend of freshly-prepared orange juice with lots of strawberries? It's one of my favorites.

LUNCH and DINNER IDEAS

Whether you're eating out or in, leafy green salads and raw soups are the high-octane fuel fare for lunch and dinner. Use your imagination, choose your favorite veggies in season, and create your own. Or choose a Level Three salad and/or raw soup from the recipe section that follows.

- Have a *Zucchini Linguini Salad!* That's right, "raw zucchini pasta," and it's really simple to make. Using a paring knife, shave long strips of organic raw zucchini, or simply use a Spirooli Spiral Slicer as outlined in the *EcoDiet* Kitchen Equipment section. Simply place your zucchini pasta in a bowl and toss it with pressed garlic, freshly chopped basil, and lots of cherry tomatoes sliced in half, all tossed with a some oil-free pesto, and served on a bed of arugula.

- If you're having lunch or dinner out, have a large Romaine lettuce salad (hold the anchovies!) with tomatoes and avocado tossed in an oil-free dressing. (I usually carry my own dressing everywhere I go…just in case!)

- How about being creative and making a bowl of raw soup and salad meal from the ingredients that you love the most?

- Summer? How about a mono fruit meal for lunch? Eat as many bananas, or mangoes, or peaches you want! Or, have an *Acai Green* or *Green and Lean Smoothie* found in the following recipe section.

- Enjoy a bowl of *Pineapple Gazpacho* soup served with a small, chopped veggie salad, tossed in your favorite oil-free dressing.

- How about a *Great Greek Salad* tonight with a bowl of *Raw Cucumber–Dill Soup?*

- If it's springtime, how about having a delicious salad bowl of your favorite greens tossed in your favorite oil-free dressing, served with a bowl of *Raw Tomato Basil Soup?*

- Or, how about a *Salsa Lettuce Wrap* with a bowl of *Gazpacho Avocado Soup?*

So let's get started! Turn the page and become familiar with the equipment and ingredients needed for your new *EcoDiet* kitchen. Then, begin this delectable *EcoDiet* journey with me—a path that is guaranteed to move you towards a long, vibrant life, and a higher state of spiritual and emotional well-being!

SETTING UP YOUR *ECODIET* KITCHEN

The following lists include the items you'll need to begin your new *EcoDiet* lifestyle. If your budget doesn't allow for a complete kitchen makeover all at once, start with the basics like a high-powered juicer and a blender that has enough RPMs to turn a handful of nuts into a creamy sauce or frozen fruit into a delicious sorbet. Then, when that special occasion rolls around, simply ask for a great food processor, and a new set of ceramic knives. Setting up your kitchen for success is simple and fun. Let's start with the basic equipment. See the *Resources* section for recommendations on where to shop for these items.

Equipment

Juicer

Health advocates everywhere agree that the single most essential piece of equipment for a whole foods organic kitchen is a high-quality juicer. My favorite is the Hurom Slow Juicer. The Hurom Slow Juicer is manufactured using state-of-the-art technology. Based on the powerful auger juicer style, this super-efficient unit uses a low-speed process to crush then press foods for increased yield with minimum waste. The extracted juice is loaded with antioxidants and vitamins, and free of foam, froth, or separation. This juicer also maximizes nutrition and taste of juiced fruits, vegetables, and grasses with its dual-stage extraction power. Best of all, it is self-cleaning! No more taking the machine apart, cleaning each part, and then putting it back together. All you have to do is pour in a cup of water, turn the juicer on, and in a few minutes you can start juicing again. Quiet and compact, the Hurom Slow Juicer can easily be left on a kitchen counter, so it's ready to go at any time.

Blender

Most health advocates would also agree that the other most essential piece of equipment for a whole foods kitchen is a high-quality blender. My favorite is the Blendtec. Most other blenders found in department stores just don't have the power to turn hard nuts into a cream sauce or cold vegetables into a warm steamy soup. This high-performance blender has the power to make whole-food juice, sprouted nut butters, fruit smoothies, sorbets, ice cream, and baby food. The Blendtec has predesigned cycle settings. When a cycle button is pushed, it automatically speeds up and slows down, then shuts off when the cycle is complete. The Blendtec Total Blender has so much power (1500 Watts) it turns ice to snow and actually comes with an ice-crushing 8-year factory warranty.

Food Processor

Throughout the years, the food processor has become the most popular kitchen appliance among gourmets everywhere. The Cuisinart PowerPrep is a professional grade food processor that outperforms any other food processor known. It dices, slices, chops, juliennes, minces, shreds, blends, purées—you name it; it does it. The name Cuisinart is synonymous with superior quality and innovation. The 14-cup PowerPrep Plus Food Processor is Cuisinart's new model. It boasts an alternate speed for dough mixing. If you are cooking for several people, the Cuisinart PowerPrep will save you time in food preparation. You will find it of help in preparing the recipes included in this book.

Spiralo Slicer and Spirooli

Designed and imported from Germany, these vertical-turning slicers create streams of raw vegetable spaghetti from zucchini, squash, and various other hard vegetables in minutes. The interchangeable blade system is fast, safe, and easy to use, and the sturdy suction legs hold securely to your kitchen counter. Just insert your vegetable and away you go. It's fast, easy, and fun to use. The kids love it! But use caution; the blades are sharp. The Spiralo Slicer stands vertically while the Spirooli is horizontal. They are the same tool with a different structure. You choose!

Sprouting Jars

Sprouting or soaking grains, beans, nuts, and seeds is fun and easy and there are two economical ways to grow sprouts. First, there is the glass jar version that can be purchased at most health food stores in various sizes. I like the half-gallon jars with strainer lids as the perfect-sized medium for growing sprouts: not too small, not too large. Wide-mouth mason jars can also be used with a lid made of a piece of cheesecloth secured with a thick rubber band. Simply place the amount needed into the jar, fill with water, let soak overnight, then drain and rise several times over the next few days.

Bulk Foods

Air-sealed glass jars are useful for storing bulk foods like grains, beans, nuts, seeds, snacks, and dried fruits. Depending on the size of your family, you'll want to purchase between fifteen and twenty jars. For convenience and easy storage, I prefer the glass square ones with pull-off or screw tops. Snack foods, such as nuts and dried fruit, and raw cane sugar and salt are best stored in the pull-off top jars sitting on your countertop for quick and easy access. Screw top jars are best for longer storage items such as beans and grains in the cupboard. If your budget is low, don't fret. These jars can even be found at most dollar stores.

LEVEL ONE
PANTRY ITEMS

Organic Grains

Quinoa	Jasmine	Forbidden rice	Short Grain Rice
Long Grain Rice	Brown Rice	Pasta	

Organic Beans

Mung Beans	Lentils	Adzuki Beans
Black Beans	Fava Beans	Butter Beans
Garbanzo Beans	Cannellini Beans	Lima Beans
Navy Beans	Kidney Beans	Pinto Beans

When stocking your pantry, be sure to always have Eden organic canned beans on hand!

Organic Miscellaneous Items

Raw Coconut Oil	Cold-pressed Olive Oil

LEVEL ONE AND TWO
PANTRY ITEMS

Organic Miscellaneous Items

Celtic Sea Salt	Vanilla Extract	Herbs and Spices
Capers	Artichoke Hearts	Sun-dried Tomatoes
Roasted Red Bell Peppers	Apple Cider Vinegar	Sweet Relish
Brown rice syrup	Brown rice vinegar	Ume Plum Vinegar
Bragg Liquid Aminos	Bragg fat-free dressings	

LEVEL ONE, TWO, AND THREE
PANTRY ITEMS

Organic Nuts

Raw almonds	Macadamia	Walnuts	Pine nuts
Pecans	Hazelnuts		

Organic Seeds

Pumpkin seeds	Sunflower seeds	Hempseeds
Chia seeds	Flaxseeds	

Organic Dried Fruit

Raisins Currants Cranberries Medjool Dates

Organic Super Foods

Green Powder Blend	Gogi berries	Gogi Powder
Acai Powder	Maca Root Powder	Carob Powder
Active Manuka Honey +16	Bee Pollen	Royal Jelly

Organic Miscellaneous Items

Raw Almond Butter	Raw Tahini	Raw olives
Raw Honey	Raw Coconut Water*	Raw Coconut Vinegar
Raw Coconut Aminos		

Harmless Harvest makes organic raw coconut water that has never been heated! If your health food doesn't carry this brand, ask them to order you a discounted case! It's absolutely delicious!

ECODIET

Recipes

The recipes in this section have been designed over the many years I owned my own gourmet vegetarian restaurant and taught hundreds of whole food preparation classes. While there are a few bottled oil-free organic salad dressings in the health food stores to have on hand in your pantry, I have included several easy-to-prepare, absolutely delicious oil-free salad dressings in the recipe section that will increase your desire to eat more leafy greens.

The key is to keep two or three of your favorites on hand, ready to whip out when you're in a fast-food hurry and need to quickly transform that ordinary plate of leafy greens into a 5-star gourmet salad.

The same holds true with sauces. You can almost always find a fresh supply of dairy and oil-free pesto in my refrigerator. In the past, whenever I would come home from an all-day outing tired and wanting to prepare something quick and easy, yet delicious, I simply cooked up (on very low heat) a medium-size serving of organic brown rice pasta, tossed it with pesto, and served it up on a huge bed of arugula greens and voila, the perfect Level One combo. But now that my taste buds desire a more Level Three raw food fare, I simply put my Spirooli to work and make myself a large plate of raw zucchini noodles and toss.

Making foods can be easy and fun! Trust me, after years of experimentation, you are getting some of my finest and most favorite recipes. I recognize that time is of the essence, so I've made great taste as simple as possible. The terrific thing is that I get so much help from Mother Nature!

Bon appétit!

LET'S GET JUICED!
Level One, Two, and Three

The Alkalizer

8 carrots
2 stalks celery
½ bunch parsley
½ bunch watercress
½ bunch spinach

Juice.

Liver/Gallbladder Cleanser

6 carrots
2 granny smith apples

Juice.

Gallbladder Cleanser

3-4 apples
1 large beetroot
1 whole lemon
1-inch piece ginger
½ jalapeño pepper

Juice.

Liver Cleanser

2 apples
2 beets
7 celery stalks
6 carrots
1-inch piece of ginger

Juice.

Intestinal Booster

1 bunch spinach
8 carrots

Juice.

Clean, Green, and Lean

½ bunch spinach
¼ head leaf lettuce
3 stalks celery
1 cucumber
2 kale leaves

Juice.

SUPERFOOD SMOOTHIES
Level One, Two, and Three

Maca Momma

2 Thai coconuts (or 16 ounces raw coconut water)
1 pineapple
2 bananas
½ cup macadamia nuts
1 tablespoon maca root powder

Open coconuts. Pour coconut water into a blender. Spoon out all the meat and place it into the blender. Blend on high speed until smooth. Add the remaining ingredients and blend on high speed again until creamy smooth. For convenience, feel free to use 16 ounces of coconut water found at most health food stores.

"Bee" Always Young

1 Thai coconut (or 16 ounces raw coconut water)
1 banana
1 teaspoon royal jelly
1 tablespoon bee pollen
2 tablespoons UMF Active Manuka honey +16
1 tablespoon maca root powder
1 teaspoon raw carob powder
½ teaspoon cinnamon powder

Open coconut. Pour coconut water into a blender. Spoon out all the meat and place it into the blender. Blend on high speed until smooth. Add the remaining ingredients and blend on high speed again until creamy smooth. For convenience, feel free to use 16 ounces of coconut water found at most health food stores.

Seeds of Change

1 cup apple or orange juice
½ banana
½ cup blueberries
1 tablespoon acai powder
2 tablespoons hempseeds
1 tablespoon chia seeds

Place all of the ingredients into a blender and blend on high speed until smooth.

Acai Green

1 banana
2 oranges, peeled
¼ cup acai juice
2 tablespoons green powder

Place all of the ingredients into a blender and blend on high speed until smooth.

Carob Malt Smoothie

1 Thai coconut (or 16 ounces raw coconut water)
1 small banana
¼ cup pumpkin seeds
2 tablespoons raw carob powder
1 tablespoon maca root powder
2 tablespoons Active Manuka honey
¼ teaspoon cinnamon
Dash of cayenne pepper

Pour coconut water into a blender. Spoon out all the meat, place it into the blender, and blend on high speed until smooth. Add the remaining ingredients and blend on high speed again until smooth. For convenience, feel free to use 16 ounces of coconut water found at most health food stores.

FRUIT SMOOTHIES
Level One, Two, and Three

Banana Date

2 cups water
1 banana
5 Medjool dates, pitted
1 tablespoon alcohol-free vanilla extract

Place all of the ingredients into a blender and blend on high speed until smooth.

Berry Good

3 oranges, juiced
1 banana
1 cup blueberries
1 cup strawberries
1 cup raspberries

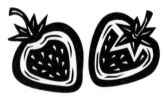

Place all of the ingredients into a blender and blend on high speed until smooth.

Tropical Delight

1 cup raw coconut water
1 large mango, diced
1 banana
1 small papaya

Place all of the ingredients into a blender and blend on high speed until smooth.

GREEN SMOOTHIES
Level One, Two, and Three

Green and Lean

16 ounces water
2 heaping cups spinach leaves
2 pears, stemmed
1 banana

In a blender, combine water, spinach, pears, and banana. Blend on the highest speed until smooth.

Dandelion Smoothie

16 ounces water or raw coconut water
1-2 cups dandelion greens, chopped
1-2 pears, chopped
2 dates, remove pit

In a blender, combine coconut water, pears, dates, and dandelion. Blend on the highest speed until smooth.

Pineapple Coconut Watercress

1 cup raw coconut water
½ pineapple, juiced
½ pineapple, diced
1 bunch watercress
1 banana

In a blender, combine pineapple juice, diced pineapple, watercress, banana, and coconut water and blend on high speed until smooth.

FRUIT SALADS
Level One, Two, and Three

Banana Date Salad

5 bananas, peeled and mashed
3 red apples, sliced in half, cored, and julienned
Honey Date Sauce
1 teaspoon cinnamon

In a medium-size bowl, place bananas. Mash them with a wide-prong fork, leaving some bite-size pieces. Top with apples. Pour desired amount of *Honey Date Sauce* over the top, then sprinkle with cinnamon and serve.

Honey Date Sauce

1 cup honey dates, sliced in half and pitted
1 cup water

In a blender, combine the dates and water and blend on high speed until smooth.

Better Than Waldorf Salad

4 Fuji apples, peeled and cut into small pieces
3 stalks celery, sliced in half and finely diced top half (saving the bottom half for garnish)
1 cup red grapes, sliced in half and seeded
1 cup Medjool dates, sliced in half, pitted, and cut into small pieces
1 cup raw walnut pieces
Honey Lemon Sauce

In a large bowl, combine apples, celery, grapes, dates, and walnuts. Toss with desired amount of *Honey Lemon Sauce* on next page. Divide equally into three tall serving bowls. Cut the remaining celery halfway down the stalk into five fanlike slices. Bottom half can be used for a spoon.

Honey Lemon Sauce

1 whole lemon, unpeeled
¼ cup Manuka honey
¼ cup water

In a blender, combine the lemon, honey, and water and blend on high speed until smooth.

Orange 'U Special Salad

3 oranges, peeled and cut into 1-inch cubes
2 avocados, sliced in half, pitted, cut into cubes, and spooned out
½ cup red onion, sliced in ½ slivers
1 package mixed salad greens
Orange Honey Sauce

In a large bowl, combine the oranges, avocados, onion, and salad greens. Pour desired amount of *Orange Honey Sauce* over the salad then toss and serve.

Orange Honey Sauce

1 orange, juiced
½ lime, juiced
1 tablespoon raw honey
1 cup cilantro leaves
1 garlic clove, peeled
1 small piece of fresh ginger

In a blender, combine the orange, lime juice, honey, cilantro, garlic, ginger, and blend on high speed until creamy smooth.

RAW SOUPS, SALADS, AND WRAPS
Level One, Two, and Three

Gazpacho Avocado Soup

3 vine-ripe tomatoes, sliced in half
1 cucumber, peeled, sliced in half, seeded, and chopped
1 green bell pepper, sliced in half, seeded, and chopped
½ red onion, peeled, quartered, and thinly sliced
2 garlic cloves, peeled and minced
1 cup parsley, stemmed and finely chopped
1 jalapeño pepper, sliced in half, seeded, and minced
1 lemon, juiced
2 avocados, halved, pitted, sliced into cubes and spooned out

Using a food processor or blender, pulse the tomatoes, cucumbers, bell peppers, onions, garlic, parsley, jalapeño pepper, and lemon juice several times, or until chopped. Transfer to a large bowl and add avocado as a delicious, and very untraditional, bite-size garnish.

Tomato Basil Soup

6 vine-ripened tomatoes, sliced in half
1 cup basil leaves, chopped
½ cup yellow onion, chopped
1 celery stalk, chopped
1 avocado, sliced in half, pitted, cut into cubes, and spooned out
1 tablespoon raw coconut aminos
1 dash cayenne pepper
1 lime, juiced

In a blender, pulse all of the above ingredients 3 to 4 times, or until chunky-smooth. Transfer to a large serving bowl and garnish with basil leaves.

Note: raw coconut aminos are available online or at your health food store.

Pineapple Gazpacho Soup

4 cups pineapple, chopped
4 cups cucumber, peeled and chopped
3–4 tablespoons jalapeño peppers, minced
4 tablespoons scallions, thinly sliced mostly white part
2 tablespoons lime juice
1 cup fresh pineapple juice
1 cup cilantro leaves
1 avocado, pitted and chopped

In a blender, purée 3 cups pineapple, 3 cups cucumber, jalapeño peppers, scallions, lime juice, and pineapple juice. Add the remaining pineapple, cucumber, and cilantro. Pulse the blender quickly a few times—the gazpacho should remain chunky. Stir in the avocado. Delicious!

Thai Coconut Soup

4 Thai coconuts
1 lime, juiced
3 tablespoons raw coconut aminos
1 tablespoon minced ginger
2 garlic cloves
½ tablespoon curry powder
1 teaspoon crushed red peppers
6 Medjool dates, pitted

In a blender, blend coconut water with coconut meat on high speed until creamy smooth, which should give you approximately 40 ounces of coconut milk. Add lime juice, raw coconut aminos, ginger, garlic cloves, curry powder, crushed red peppers, and blend. Taste your soup and adjust according to your personal flavor buds! Add pitted dates and pulse several times, leaving small bits of dates. Divide among four bowls; add the garnish ingredients listed below to the center of each bowl, and top with a few cilantro leaves.

Garnish

2 cups heirloom cherry tomatoes, quartered
1 cucumber, peeled, seeded, and diced
½ red bell pepper, cut into very thin slivers
½ cup cilantro leaves

Great Greek Salad

2 large cucumbers, peeled, cut in half lengthwise, seeds scooped out, and cut into crescent moons
3 bell peppers (a combination of green and red), cut in halves, seeds removed, and cut into ½-inch rounds
1 small red onion, cut into thin crescents
2 vine-ripe tomatoes, cut into quarters
⅓ cup raw Greek olives
½ cup fresh or dried dill weed
2 tablespoons fresh or dried Greek oregano
1 lemon, juiced

In a large bowl, combine cucumbers, bell peppers, onion, tomatoes, olives, dill weed, and oregano then toss with lemon juice.

Italian Kale Salad

1 large bunch kale, ribs removed and finely chopped
3 cloves garlic, pressed
2 dashes cayenne pepper
½ lemon, juiced
1 large avocado, halved, pitted, cut into cubes, and spooned out
¼ cup nutritional yeast
½ cup raw kalamata olives, pitted
½ cup sun-dried tomatoes, cut into small pieces
¼ cup pine nuts

In a large salad bowl, place the kale, garlic, cayenne pepper, ½ avocado, and lemon juice. Massage the ingredients for about 2 minutes or until the kale begins to wilt and release some moisture. Add the remaining avocado, nutritional yeast, olives, sun-dried tomatoes, and gently toss with your hands. Add the pine nuts, toss again, and serve.

Winter Root Salad

1 fresh beetroot, peeled and julienned
1 large carrot, peeled and julienned
½ celery root, peeled and julienned
1 fennel bulb, sliced very thin
1 Fuji apple, cored and diced
½ a small radicchio head, cut into small pieces
1 large handful baby arugula
Apple Juice Dressing

Slice the beetroots, carrots, and celery root with a mandolin or in a food processor into julienne strips and then place in a large mixing bowl. Add the fennel, apple, radicchio, and arugula. Toss with *Apple Juice Dressing*, garnish with sprigs of fennel leaves, and serve.

Apple Juice Dressing

1 apple, juiced
1 lemon, juiced
1 tablespoon raw honey
2 tablespoons hempseeds
1 tablespoon chia seeds

Whisk until smooth and serve.

Watercress Papaya Salad

1-2 ripe papayas, seeded and sliced (about 1 quart)
5 cups watercress sprigs
½ cup Vidalia onion, thinly sliced
Sweet and Sour Dressing

In the center of a wide, shallow glass bowl, mound papayas and onion; toss with *Sweet and Sour Dressing*; spread the watercress around the sides, and then drizzle with more dressing.

Sweet and Sour Dressing

2 lemons, juiced
1 tablespoon raw honey
1 tablespoon poppy seeds
2 tablespoons minced fresh mint leaves
½ teaspoon ground coriander

Whisk until smooth, pour over papaya salad, and serve.

Zucchini Linguini Pesto Salad

4 firm medium-size zucchini, spiraled
1 cup basil pesto or marinara sauce
¼ cup sun-dried tomatoes, diced
Fresh basil leaves

To make long noodles out of zucchini, simply use a vegetable spiral slicer like the Spiralo or Spirooli. To improve the texture of the noodles, try making them about six hours before serving, allowing them to sit in an uncovered bowl at room temperature. When noodles are ready, toss with pesto and sun-dried tomatoes or raw marinara sauce. Place it in your favorite bowl, then garnish with basil leaves.

Oil-Free Pesto

1 cup pine nuts
⅔ cup water
4 garlic cloves, peeled
2 cups packed basil leaves, stemmed

In a blender, combine the pine nuts and water and blend on high speed until creamy smooth. Add the garlic and pulse for approximately 1 minute. Be sure not to over-blend, as you want a semi-nutty consistency: not too smooth, not too chunky. Add basil leaves and continue to pulse until the basil can be seen only as tiny flakes. Store in a sealed airtight glass container like a mason jar in your refrigerator until ready to use.

Fig Fuji Salsa Wrap

2 Fuji apples, peeled, sliced in half, cored, and diced
1 cup fresh figs, sliced into quarter pieces
½ cup red onion, finely chopped
1 cup green bell pepper, finely chopped
1 tablespoon fresh ginger, grated
1 serrano chile, sliced in half, seeded, and finely chopped
½ cup roasted, spicy piñata pumpkin seeds
1 lime, juiced
1 head leafy green lettuce, separate leaves (optional)

In a large bowl, combine the apples, figs, onion, bell pepper, ginger, serrano chile, pumpkin seeds, and lime juice, then toss. Transfer to an airtight bowl, seal, and let sit several hours before serving to give all of the flavors time to merge into a fabulously tasteful delight. Serve wrapped inside your favorite leafy green lettuce leaf.

Fruit Salsa Wrap

1 cup strawberries, stemmed and medium diced
1 cup kiwi, peeled and medium diced
1 cup banana, peeled and medium diced
1 teaspoon fresh cilantro leaves, minced
1 serrano pepper, sliced in half, seeded, and minced
1 orange, juiced
1 lime, juiced
1 head leafy green lettuce, leaves separated (optional)

In a medium-size bowl, combine the strawberries, kiwi, banana, cilantro, serrano pepper, orange juice, and lime juice, then toss. Transfer to an airtight bowl, seal, and let sit several hours before serving to give all of the flavors time to merge into a fabulously tasteful delight. Serve wrapped inside your favorite leafy green lettuce leaf.

VEGETABLE SALADS
Level One and Two

Romaine and Artichoke Salad

2 romaine hearts, stems cut off and leaves separated
1 can organic artichoke hearts, cut into quarters
2 avocados, sliced in half, pitted, cut into cubes, and spooned out
2 vine-ripened tomatoes, diced
¼ cup organic capers
Thousand Island Dressing
1 handful broccoli sprouts

On a large serving platter, arrange romaine leaves; place artichoke hearts, avocados, tomatoes, and capers in equal portions inside each leaf. Drizzle desired amount of *Thousand Island Dressing* over the top; then garnish each leaf with broccoli sprouts and serve.

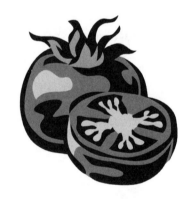

Thousand Island Dressing

2 vine-ripened tomatoes
½ cup sun-dried tomatoes
½ cup pine nuts
4 tablespoons apple cider vinegar
2 garlic cloves, peeled
¼ cup raw honey
½ cup organic sweet relish
Salt to taste

In a blender, combine tomatoes, sun-dried tomatoes, pine nuts, vinegar, garlic, honey, and salt and blend on high speed until creamy smooth. Add relish and pulse for 10 seconds.

Butter Me Up Salad

2 heads butternut lettuce
2 avocados, sliced in half, pitted, cut into cubes and spooned out
½ cup corn kernels, cut off cob
1 jalapeño pepper, minced
2 cups cilantro leaves, stemmed and minced
2 cups yellow and red bell peppers, diced
2 cups ripe tomatoes, chopped
Yogurt-Mint Dressing

In a medium-size bowl, combine avocado, jalapeño pepper, and cilantro, and toss. On a large serving platter, arrange lettuce leaves then spoon avocado mixture in equal portions into each leaf. Top each leaf with equal amounts of bell peppers, corn, and tomatoes. Drizzle each leaf with desired amounts of yogurt-mint dressing.

Yogurt-Mint Dressing

1 cup plain coconut yogurt, drained
⅓ cup fresh mint, finely chopped
1 small lemon, juiced

In a small-size glass bowl, combine yogurt, mint, and lemon juice. Whisk until blended.

Berry Good Salad

½ pound mixed salad greens
1 cup blueberries
1 cup raspberries
1 cup blackberries
1 cup strawberries
½ cup cherry tomatoes, sliced in half
1 cup raw walnuts
Red Raspberry Dressing

In a large bowl, combine salad greens, berries, tomatoes, and walnuts then toss with desired amount of *Red Raspberry Dressing* and stack in the middle of large serving platter.

Red Raspberry Dressing

⅓ cup raspberries (or organic raspberry jam)
⅓ cup water
1 tablespoon apple cider vinegar
1 tablespoon raw honey
1 garlic clove, peeled

In a blender, combine raspberries, water, vinegar, honey, and garlic and blend on high speed until well blended.

Over the Rainbow Salad

1 head romaine lettuce, cut into bite-size pieces
2 beets, julienned
1 medium carrot, julienned
1 medium diakon radish, julienned
2 medium tomatoes, diced
1 package sunflower sprouts
2 avocados, sliced in half, pitted, cut into cubes and spooned out
1 green pepper, cut into small rounds and seeded
Miso Good Dressing

In a large bowl, add lettuce then arrange beets, carrots, radish, and tomatoes in mounds of four around the periphery of the leaves. In between each mound, place a handful of sunflower sprouts and avocados. Garnish with bell pepper rounds and serve with desired amount of *Miso Good Dressing*.

Miso Good Dressing

½ cup water
1½ cups mellow miso
¼ cup apple cider vinegar
¾ cup red onion, chopped
⅓ cup raw honey

In a blender, combine water, miso, vinegar, onion, and honey and blend on high speed until smooth and creamy.

Yin Yang Salad

½ head Savoy cabbage, sliced in half and finely shredded
¼ head red cabbage, cut in quarters and finely shredded
½ carrot, julienned
1½ cups cilantro, chopped
½ cup raisins
Sweet and Sour Dressing

In a large bowl, combine cabbages, carrot, cilantro, and raisins and toss with desired amount of *Sweet and Sour Dressing.*

Sweet and Sour Dressing

¾ cup raw almond butter
½ cup water
¾ cup brown rice syrup
⅔ cup brown rice vinegar
1 tablespoon Bragg Liquid Aminos
Cayenne pepper to taste

In a blender, combine almond butter, water, brown rice syrup, brown rice vinegar, Bragg Liquid Aminos, and cayenne pepper. Blend on high speed until creamy and smooth.

Radicchio Pear Salad

2 heads Radicchio, sliced in half and finely shredded
1 head Frisse lettuce, cut off stem
2 firm pears, cored and sliced thin
2 tablespoons shallots, finely diced
⅓ cup walnuts
Creamy Almond Dressing

Place the above ingredients in a serving bowl and toss.

Creamy Almond Dressing

½ cup raw almonds, blanched
¼ cup water
3 tablespoons apple cider vinegar
2 tablespoons raw honey
1 clove garlic
½ teaspoon dried mustard

In a blender, combine almonds, water, vinegar, honey, garlic, and mustard and blend on high speed until creamy smooth. Pour dressing over the salad, toss, scatter the oregano leaves on top and serve.

HOT AND STEAMY SOUPS
Level One

Miso Good Asparagus Soup

1 bunch spring onions, diced
3 carrots, peeled, cut in half and sliced diagonally
1 pound asparagus, cut into 2-inch pieces
1 quart water
6 ounces sweet white miso

In a medium-size soup pot, cook the onions and carrots on low heat for 10 minutes in a small amount of water or vegetable broth, or until carrots are tender. In a steamer pan, steam the asparagus for 5 to 10 minutes, or until tender. Transfer the asparagus to the soup pot, then stir. In a blender, combine water and miso and blend on low speed for one minute or until thoroughly blended. Pour miso-water into soup pot and stir. Cover and cook on low heat for approximately 10 minutes. Remove from heat and let sit for 30 minutes before serving.

Black Bean Soup

1 large yellow onion, chopped
2 garlic cloves, peeled and chopped
1–2 carrots, peeled and diced
1 teaspoon salt
1 jalapeño pepper, cut in half, seeded and minced
1 teaspoon ground cumin
½ teaspoon dried oregano
½ teaspoon thyme
1 32-ounce box vegetable broth
2 cans organic black beans, drained and rinsed
1 cup fresh cilantro leaves, stemmed and chopped
2 tablespoons Bragg Liquid Aminos
1 cup spring onions, chopped
1 avocado, cut in half, pitted, cut into cubes and spooned out

In a large soup pot, cook the onion and garlic on low heat in water or vegetable broth for 10 minutes, or until onion is translucent. Add carrots, salt, jalapeño pepper, cumin, oregano, and thyme. Cook for 2 to 3 more minutes; add vegetable broth and beans. Cover and cook on low heat for 30 minutes. Remove from heat. Add ½ cup cilantro and Bragg Liquid Aminos and let sit for 30 minutes. Garnish with chopped spring onions, cilantro, and avocado.

Vegetable Bean Chili

2 16-ounce cans ground organic tomatoes
3 cups water
3 medium yellow onions, cut into bite size pieces
4 carrots, peeled and diced
3 large bell peppers (1 red, 1 green, 1 yellow)
1 tablespoon chili peppers
2–3 tablespoons chili powder
3 cans pinto beans
2½ tablespoons salt

In a large soup pot, combine tomatoes, water, onions, and carrots and cook on low heat for 10 minutes. Add bell peppers, chili peppers, and chili powder, then stir. Cook for another 10 minutes. Remove from heat. Add beans and salt. Cover and let sit for approximately 1 hour.

Roasted Red Bell Pepper Bean Soup

3 red bell peppers, cut into halves, seeded, and sliced lengthwise into ¼-inch strips
1 whole garlic bulb
1 large yellow onion, chopped
2 15-ounce cans organic Cannellini beans, drained and rinsed
1 32-ounce box vegetable broth
1 teaspoon chili peppers
2 teaspoons salt

Preheat the oven to 250°F. Place red bell peppers and garlic bulb on a baking sheet and cook for 1 hour, or until peppers are tender. Remove from the oven, set the garlic bulb aside; place peppers on a chop block, then chop. In a large skillet, lightly cook the onion in a small amount of water or vegetable broth for 10 minutes, or until onion is translucent. Remove garlic cloves from bulb. Add peppers and garlic cloves, then sauté for 2 to 3 more minutes. Add beans, vegetable broth, chili peppers, and salt, stirring for 1 minute. Cover and cook for 15 minutes on low heat. Transfer to a blender and blend on high speed until creamy smooth. Return to pot, then cover and let sit for 30 minutes.

Potato Corn Soup

1½ quarts water
4 cups yellow onion, chopped
3 cups celery, chopped
6 garlic cloves, peeled and minced
2 tablespoons Bragg Liquid Aminos
5 cups corn kernels, cut off cob
5 cups potatoes, cut into 1-inch cubes
2 tablespoons dill weed
2 teaspoons salt
¼ teaspoon black pepper

In a large soup pot, combine water, onion, and celery. Cover and cook on low heat for approximately 20 minutes. Stir in garlic and Bragg Liquid Aminos; add corn and potatoes, then cook for another 10 minutes. Remove from heat. Place one-half corn and potato mixture in a blender and blend on high speed until creamy smooth. Add dill weed, salt, and pepper, then pulse 3 to 4 times. Pour purée back into soup pot and stir with remaining soup mixture. Cover and let sit for at least 1 hour.

Potato Leek Soup

1½ quarts water
4 cups yellow onion, chopped
4 leeks, finely chopped
3 cups celery, chopped
6 garlic cloves, peeled and minced
2 tablespoons Bragg Liquid Aminos
5 cups potatoes, sliced into 1-inch cubes
2 tablespoons dill weed
2 teaspoons salt
¼ teaspoon black pepper

In a large soup pot, combine water, onion, and celery. Cover and cook on low heat for approximately 20 minutes. Stir in garlic, Bragg Liquid Aminos, and potatoes, then cook for another 10 minutes. Remove from heat. Place one-half corn and potato mixture in a blender and blend on high speed until creamy smooth. Add dill weed, salt, and pepper then pulse 3 to 4 times. Pour purée back into soup pot and stir with remaining soup mixture. Cover and let sit for at least 1 hour

Cream of Broccoli Soup

5 cups water
2 large yellow onions, chopped
1 large bunch broccoli, chopped
2 tablespoons Bragg Liquid Aminos
3 tablespoons tarragon
Salt to taste
Plum Good Cream Sauce

In a large soup pot, add water, onions, broccoli, Bragg Liquid Aminos, tarragon, and salt. Cover and cook over low heat for approximately 15 minutes. Transfer to a blender and blend on high speed until creamy smooth. Add desired amount of Plum Good Cream Sauce and blend on low speed until well blended. And it really is plum good!

Plum Good Cream Sauce

1 cup raw almonds, blanched
1 cup water
2 tablespoons Ume Plum Vinegar
1 teaspoon salt

In a blender, combine almonds, water, vinegar, and salt and blend on high speed until creamy smooth. Reserve a small amount to drizzle on top of the soup when serving.

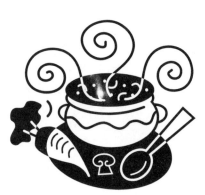

Fennel Potato Soup

¼ cup water
2 fennel bulbs, chopped
1 large onion, chopped
8 ounces Yukon gold potatoes, diced
2 cups vegetarian broth
1 teaspoon fennel seeds, finely crushed
¾ teaspoon dried tarragon
dash of salt and pepper

Add water, fennel bulbs, onions, and potatoes to a large soup pan and sauté until slightly softened, about 7 minutes. Add vegetarian broth, fennel seeds, tarragon, salt, and pepper; cover, and simmer until vegetables are very tender, about 20 minutes. Working in batches, purée soup in blender until smooth. Return soup to same pot. Simmer until flavors blend, about 5 minutes, thinning with more broth if desired.

NOW THE BIG QUESTION IS...
WHAT DO WE FEED OUR CHILDREN?

EcoDiet4Kids™

As newly converted *EcoDiet* advocates, we want to make sure our children are also eating sustainable, eco-friendly foods. But sometimes this isn't so easy. Before we changed to an organic, plant-based diet, their taste buds were already conditioned to a salty, sugary, fast-food fare, so they cried when they didn't get it. These days, most of our children's taste buds are conditioned to "fake foods" by the time they're toddlers!

Most of our children are brought up in a family in which both parents work and are often taken to daycare where they are fed a daily fare of chemically-processed foods.

Then, after coming home from a long day at work, parents are too tired to prepare a nutritious meal and want something simple, quick, and preferably inexpensive. Microwave dinners and other packaged "fake foods" loaded with toxic chemicals offer the solution to making our lives a little easier. Oftentimes we feel guilty because of our busy lifestyles and give our children whatever they want to eat, especially if it means avoiding yet another battle.

Now, childhood obesity is on the rise. The Centers for Disease Control report childhood obesity has more than tripled in the past 30 years. Currently, 12.5 million American kids ages 2 to 19 are obese—17% of the population in this age range. Another 16.5% are at risk for becoming overweight, mostly because of their unhealthy food choices.

According to the Mayo Clinic, childhood obesity is particularly troubling because the extra pounds often start children on the path to health problems that were once confined to adults, such as diabetes, high blood pressure, and high cholesterol. Childhood obesity can also lead to poor self-esteem and depression.

Dietary-related childhood diseases, such as ADD (attention deficient disorder) and ADHD (attention deficient hyperactivity disorder), are also on the rise. Most often, children are given Ritalin (a central nervous system stimulant), to make the lives of both teachers and parents easier.

Then, we learn about the huge part that the foods our children eat plays in their health and well-being. They snub their noses at the plate of organic, whole foods we eagerly place before them, push it away, and say something like "I want some real food!" Or they might come home from school and tell us they hated what was in their lunchbox, that their friends are eating potato chips, cupcakes, white bread, and peanut butter for lunch, so why can't they? Or they come home with an invitation to a friend's birthday party at an arcade-style pizza place, with all the frills and thrills of video games and rides.

So what is a parent supposed to do?

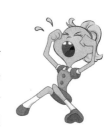

As a working parent of two, the first step I took was to increase my children's intake of fruits and vegetables. Instead of giving them white crackers with processed "fake" cheese, I'd give them sliced oranges or apples or maybe even an apple or a banana with organic, raw almond butter. Next, I started making them a fruity-green smoothie in the morning, which they loved. Then, I slowly eliminated the processed "fake foods" loaded with artificial flavors and toxic chemicals and replaced them with the organic versions from the health food store. Thankfully, the growing health industry is making healthier food choices simple and clear.

As an example, if you are a working parent, and in a hurry in the morning to get everyone off to school and don't have time to even prepare a bowl of fruit or smoothie, there are healthier alternatives. Reading labels and shifting to organics is key to transitioning your children to a more organic, whole foods lifestyle.

Even though I don't recommend cereals for an *EcoDiet*, consider the difference in the ingredients between a typical grocery store non-organic cereal and a health food store organic cereal. One is loaded with genetically modified foods, synthetic vitamins, sugar, preservatives, and artificial flavors—the other is not.

Kellogg's Corn Pops	Envirokidz Gorilla Munch
Milled corn, sugar, soluble corn fiber, molasses, salt, soybean and/or cottonseed oils, mono and diglycerides, sodium ascorbate and ascorbic acid (vitamin C), niacinamide, zinc oxide, reduced iron, wheat starch, pyridoxine hydrochloride (vitamin B6), riboflavin (vitamin B2), thiamin hydrochloride (vitamin B1), vitamin A palmitate, annatto color, BHT (preservative), folic acid, vitamin D and vitamin B12.	Organic corn meal, organic evaporated cane juice, sea salt.

If you're making your child toast for breakfast or a sandwich for their school lunchbox, consider the difference in the ingredients between typical grocery store bread and an organic, health-food-store organic bread. Again, one is loaded with genetically modified foods, synthetic vitamins, sugar, preservatives, and artificial flavors—the other is not.

Wonder Enriched Bread	Ezekiel 4:9™ Sprouted Bread
Enriched wheat flour, barley malt, ferrous sulfate (iron), B vitamins (niacin, thiamin, mononitrate (B1), riboflavin (B2), folic acid), high fructose corn syrup, potato flour, yeast, buttermilk; contains 2% or less of: wheat gluten, dough conditioners (potassium bromate, sodium, stearoyl lactylate, alpha amylase), soy flour, calcium carbonate, monoglycerides, monocalcium phosphate, calcium sulfate, calcium propionate (to retain freshness).	Organic sprouted wheat*, organic sprouted barley*, organic sprouted millet*, malted barley*, organic sprouted lentils*, organic sprouted soybeans*, organic spelt*, filtered water, fresh yeast, sea salt.

*Organically grown and processed in accordance with the California organic foods act of 1990.

The following are a few ideas your children may enjoy for breakfast, lunch, and dinner. You may also find more recipes they'll enjoy in the recipe section.

BREAKFAST

If you are preparing your children's breakfast on-the-go, take a few minutes to prepare any of these healthy ecotarian breakfasts. They are all loaded with fiber, fruit, and protein. Your kids will love it too, especially if you top their dish with a handful of raisins for a bit of sweetness.

- Fruit slices or berries with coconut yogurt
- Granola with berries and almond milk
- Organic cereal (let them pick it out) with bananas and almond milk
- Toasted sprouted bread with Turkish fig spread (blend Turkish figs, chia seeds, and water)
- Fruit smoothie
- Oatmeal with honey, almond milk, and raisins
- Sprouted bagel with organic, raw almond butter

LUNCH

Far from the heavy, starchy lunches our kids may be used to, several small, snack-like servings with a variety of foods are the two keys to creating a healthy lunch for your children. And it's easy. Many lunch foods can be prepared in advance and in large quantities for your children's lunchboxes. Each morning, simply fill up several small containers with a variety of food items.

Quick organic lunchbox food suggestions would include several of these items, depending upon your child's taste buds and appetite:

- Fresh fruit, sliced or whole
- Dried fruit
- Trail mix
- Popcorn
- Raw crackers with raw macadamia nut butter
- Applesauce or fruit cup
- Sprouted bread with raw almond butter and organic jelly
- Vegetable wraps
- Carrot sticks or mini pita breads with bean dip or hummus

DINNER

One of the organic, whole foods my kids asked for first was organic hummus. Its creamy texture and vibrant flavors were a mouth-watering pleasure for them. It's easy to make and stays fresh for more than a week, so you don't have to worry about having a healthy protein on hand that your kids will love (even though it will probably be eaten before the week is up). Other eco-friendly kid-dinner ideas are:

- Sprouted hummus and baked blue tortilla chips with a finely chopped salad
- Baked "fries" with their favorite steamed veggies
- Vegetable or bean soup (see soup recipes)
- Rice, millet, or quinoa and your child's favorite veggies
- Sprouted tortilla pizza crust topped with lots of fresh vegetables and almond cheese

- Baked potatoes with steamed broccoli
- Organic brown rice pasta with organic, sugar-free tomato sauce

However, for you and your children to move into the highest state of health and well-being possible, always remember that grains and beans are transitional foods. The two most important *EcoDiet* ingredients are fruits and vegetables—the alkalizers of the body.

Fruits are number one and vegetables are number two!

PLANT EATER BEWARE!

Eating lots of colorful fruits and vegetables filled with phytonutrients is very addictive. This is because we are plant eaters by design. Like breath awareness and sunbathing, once you start eating the way nature intended, there's no turning back. If you're not careful, you may begin to feel so good you'll have to stop taking all those drugs you've been taking. So beware! If you're not ready to live in an alkaline, oxygen-rich, slim, bronzed, healthy body then you may want to think twice before eating all of those fruits and vegetables: they help maintain high oxygen levels!

ECODIET FUEL GROUP #2—AIR

FUEL YOUR BODY THROUGH THE POWER OF YOUR BREATH

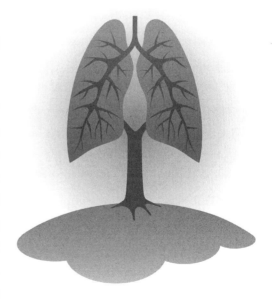

As we evolve out of the acidic "ash" of dietary devolution up through the previously prescribed three levels towards a more 100% raw vegan diet, we must come face-to-face with this fact: food is an acquired habit, just like smoking and drinking. Now I know this is "a lot to swallow," but it's a fact! Our body is a microcosm of the macrocosm we call the

Universe. Every cell in our body, and there are trillions of them, is made up of millions of atoms, each being a miniature solar system with "planets" in the form of electrons orbiting them.

Consider this for a moment: The solar system doesn't eat food for nourishment. Neither do electrons or atoms or cells. So why should we? Our body took form from one single cell called the mother cell that gave birth to trillions of daughter cells. A cell is close to being a duplicate of a water droplet, and recall that water is made of 90% oxygen.

So why not move up the acidic dietary devolution scale, eat less, breathe more, and live longer!

OXYGEN IS THE KEY TO LIFE!

While we can't see it, taste it, or touch it, air is our most vital nutrient. When you consider that our bodies are made up of 65% oxygen, it's easy to wrap our minds around the fact that our health problems, often undiagnosed, can often be traced back to shallow breathing, which results in a lack of oxygen.

Like the wind that circulates air throughout our planet's atmosphere, our breath circulates the air we breathe throughout our internal atmosphere, cleansing, feeding, alkalizing, and oxygenating every cell of our body. In fact, when we learn to breathe properly, our breath has the power to eliminate acids and alkalize us like nothing else. With the sheer movement of breathing out carbon dioxide (an acidic compound), our blood is alkalized and oxygenized.

Yet today, we remain unaware that our breath—and specifically conscious breathing—is a critical key to optimum health, a long life, and an overall state of well-being.

We have become a nation of stress-driven, sedentary, shallow-chest breathers. Most of us are taking a minimal amount of breath into our lungs, generally by drawing air into the top of the lungs (chest area) using the intercostals muscle instead of through the full length of the lungs using the diaphragm. We don't realize that 80% of the oxygen exchange between the lungs and the blood occurs at the bottom of the lungs. So, those of us who are breathing shallowly throughout the day are not getting enough oxygen. We are also unaware of the consequences of this—a build-up of carbon dioxide in the blood, and the acidification of the body.

However, if we take the time to focus on our breath every day and learn how to breathe correctly—that is, taking long, full breaths through our diaphragm—our breath has the power to turn most ecological breakdowns around. Our breath is truly the breath of life. It is our miracle!

Consider this:

- Science has proven that cancer is anaerobic; it does not survive at high levels of oxygenation. Otto Warburg proved that oxygen levels were low and carbon dioxide (CO_2) levels were elevated in cancer patients.
- Shortness of breath and heart disease are directly linked—the heart goes into spasm when it is deprived of oxygen.
- Studies have shown that there is a high correlation between high blood pressure and poor breathing.
- Optimal breathing helps to promote weight loss; oxygen burns fat and calories.
- Breathing well is the key to sleeping well and waking up feeling rested.
- Virtually every health condition and human activity is improved with optimal breathing.
- Clinical studies prove that oxygenation, wellness, and life span are totally dependent on proper diaphragmatic breathing.
- Lung volume (the percentage of air that the lungs can hold at any given time) is a primary marker for how long you will live.

DIAPHRAGM BREATHING

The great news is that with conscious breathing, you can adjust and regulate a host of chemical and biological factors that are vital to your overall health, life span, and well-being. In fact, many medical symptoms and disease conditions can be improved and even healed with slow, full breaths, which is experienced through deep, full inhalations and long, slow exhalations using your diaphragm.

The diaphragm is a muscular wall below the rib cage that acts as a natural partition between our heart and lungs and the lower organs. When we take a full, deep breath, the diaphragm moves through its entire range downward to massage and oxygenate the liver, stomach, and other organs and tissues below it. It then squeezes upward to massage and oxygenate the heart.

Also, when we take in a full deep breath the diaphragm moves farther down into the abdomen, assisting our lungs to expand more completely into the chest cavity. This means that with each breath, more oxygen is taken in and more carbon dioxide is eliminated. It also means that with each full, deep breath, we're increasing blood flow and peristalsis and pumping the lymph more efficiently throughout our lymphatic system. The lymphatic system, an important part of our immune system associated with cleansing and elimination, has no means of pumping the lymph fluids other than muscular movements, including the movements of breathing.

When the mind is focused on the breath and the nervous system is calm, there is less stress on the body and we experience better digestion and elimination. Fewer, fuller breaths also help to reduce your appetite and keep your emotions and senses under control. So, rather than getting trapped in a frenetic, high-energy chest-breathing pattern, emulate the slower, deeper habits of the giant tortoise and work to take four to six breaths per minute.

Want to eliminate stress?
BREATHE!

No matter what your present stresses may be, whether it be mental, physical or emotional, breath awareness can assist you in turning them around. Your breath is the key to becoming aware of unconscious emotional impulses and knee-jerk reactions that may be playing out in your life. Every trauma you've ever had influences the way you breathe. When breathing isn't full and deep, it's an indication that muscular tension has been created by conscious or subconscious trauma. When we have unresolved issues, mental tension causes the breath to become shallow and tight, which inevitably acidifies and deoxygenizes you.

Your breath is the wave that connects your body, mind, and emotions. By simply becoming aware of your breath and how you are breathing, especially when negative or limiting thoughts, painful feelings, or destructive behaviors arise, many wonderful changes occur.

Observe your breath right now. With mouth closed, feel the sensations of your breath as it moves in and out of your nostrils. Take a few minutes and explore the subtle details and sensations you may be feeling.

Breathe.

Let your whole body relax and soften. Feel yourself (all of you) soften—your body, your mind, and your emotions. Notice how relaxed and slow your breathing becomes, just with focused attention.

Breathe.

When your breath enters the inner nasal cavity, it stimulates the first cranial nerve, resulting in vivid mental images.

Breathe.

With continued deep breathing, even childhood traumas and other repressed emotions are released. Regular deep-breathing practice over time blows out the mental modifiers that distort conscious awareness. Thus, no matter what physical symptoms or psychological challenges you may be experiencing, if you focus your attention on your breath and feed from this bread of life every day with a grateful heart while asking for whatever it is that you need. I believe in time all of your needs will be met.

Breath awareness and focused intention is the key.

Want a slim, trim body?
BREATHE!

Deep breathing greatly assists in facilitating weight loss due to the fact that large amounts of oxygen cause the chemical reactions in your body to take place much faster; this is what aerobic exercise does, and this is what creates a high (fast) metabolism. Thus, you burn more calories than you take in and burn more body fat. In a relatively short time you'll not only feel the difference, you'll see the difference.

The answer is to simply breathe long, slow, full breaths and do it often throughout the day. Whenever you feel stressed, redirect your breath and breathe. If stress isn't managed properly, your body will burn glycogen (the main way the body stores glucose for later use) instead of fat, for that extra energy needed. Just by triggering a relaxation response with a few deep breaths, your body is encouraged to burn fat instead.

Want to live longer?
BREATHE!

Did you know that certain species that breathe fewer times a minute tend to live longer than species that breathe a comparably greater number of times per minute? A giant tortoise takes only about four breaths a minute. An elephant takes only four to five breaths a minute, and when resting, an alligator may take only one breath a minute. Though elephants and alligators don't live quite as long as a giant tortoise, they're certainly on the high end of life spans in the animal kingdom. Dogs, as well as other animals like cats and mice, take many more breaths a minute and live a decidedly shorter period of time.

Human beings, however, exist somewhere in between the dogs and the giant tortoises in both life span and breaths per minute. Humans tend to take between twelve and twenty breaths a minute, and they tend to live between 60 to 100 years.

It's interesting to note that for these species that the range of breaths per minute is proportionally similar to that of the range of expected life span.

While there are many programs, tonics, and marketable systems that promise greater longevity, if you will simply learn to take slow, full breaths through your diaphragm, you will increase your life span—and the great thing is that it won't cost you a penny.

The key is daily practice!

TRANSFORMATIONAL BREATHING EXERCISES

Learning to develop the transformational power of your breath is of the utmost importance. It is an indispensable aid to superior health, peak performance, managing stress, and life extension. It can also help you to burn those extra, unwanted pounds. Like me, if you find it's tough to exercise on a regular basis, try a few deep-breathing exercises, which can be done anytime, anywhere.

The following seven deep-breathing exercises can be performed sitting down or standing up. I call these breathing exercises breathercise®.

So if you're ready, let's try a few.

Breathercise #1

Sit comfortably with eyes open or shut. With mouth closed, inhale and exhale several times. Next, begin slowly exhaling through your nose, counting to seven, starting at the top of your chest, moving down through your mid-torso and into your diaphragm. (Remember that the diaphragm is located just below the sternum in the V formed by the rib cage.) Pause for seven counts. Begin inhaling slowly through your nose, counting to seven, starting at your diaphragm, expanding your belly, then your mid-torso, and lastly the top of your chest. Pause for seven counts and exhale as before. Repeat 5–10 times.

Breathercise #2

Combine breathing with intention. As you inhale you can think, "I am healthy, whole, and complete," and as you exhale you can think, "I am loving, forgiving, and compassionate." Or, as you inhale you can think, "I am one with God—God is the breath that breathes me," and as you exhale think, "God is my source." I invite you to create your own positive thoughts and affirmations and watch as you breathe them into reality.

Breathercise #3

Combine breathing with movement. As you slowly breathe in and expand, allow your hands and arms to express this expansion. Allow your body to move in some way, in sync with the breathing. You can also breathe in rhythm to your footsteps as you walk or run. A beautiful exercise is to sit, and as you breathe in, arch your back and lift your head. As you breathe out, lower your chin and curl your spine.

Breathercise #4

Breathe to slim down. While sitting or standing, begin by blowing all of the air out of your lungs through your mouth. When you feel as though you don't have any more air to expel, give it one more thrust, completely emptying your lungs. Relax for a few seconds. Close your mouth and quickly inhale through your nose, pulling as much air into your lungs as possible, always focusing your breath onto the area of the diaphragm. As the diaphragm expands, the lower abdomen should rise slightly, followed by the chest. Continue to steadily pull the air in as deeply as you can, completely filling your lungs.

When you feel as if you've taken in all the air you can, open your mouth and take a final gasp of air in through your mouth. Hold for 7–10 seconds. Open your mouth wide and exhale from the diaphragm with a quick, explosive breath through your mouth. Again, you should breathe out hard enough that you are able to hear the sound of your breath as you force the air from deep inside. Continue exhaling, completely emptying your lungs. As you blow the air out, roll your stomach in and up. This is the most important step, particularly if you want to flatten your stomach, tone your abdominal muscles, and oxygenate every cell of your body.

Breathercise #5

One of my favorite deep-breathing exercises is rebounding on a mini-trampoline. It's easy to fit it into your daily routine. I often rebound several times a day while watching Oprah or listening to music. Some scientists have even concluded that jumping on a mini-trampoline is one of the most effective exercises yet devised by humans, especially because of the effect rebounding has on the lymph system. The lymph fluid moves through channels called vessels that are filled with one-way valves, so the lymph always moves in the same direction. The main lymph vessels run up the legs, up the arms, and up the torso. This is why the vertical up-and-down movement of rebounding is so effective to pump the lymph.

The mini-trampoline subjects the body to gravitational pulls ranging from zero at the top of each bounce to 2–3 times the force of gravity at the bottom, depending on how high a person is rebounding. This gravitational pull pumps the lymph like nothing else. Then, when you add harmonizing, deep-breaths to your rebounding bounce, the alkalizing effect goes off the chart.

Breathercise #6

Breathe rapidly to massage your organs. Sit in a comfortable position. With mouth closed, use your belly to force air in and out through your nose as fast and equally as possible. Continue for 10–15 seconds at first, and then as you become more accustomed to this type of rapid breath, increase it to one full minute. This breath practice is an ancient belly breath that energizes while toning the abdomen and massaging the internal organs and lymph system. This type of breathing activates the lungs, neck, chest, and abdomen.

Breathercise #7

Breathe a rebirthing circular breath. The idea of circular breathing is to make the inhale active and the exhale passive and to connect each breath without pauses. Rebirthing breathwork is a technique that assists in releasing and healing suppressed emotions such as anger, fear, and sadness. It is a powerful tool in overcoming psychological trauma, such as birth trauma, as well as improving personal energy and conscious awareness. If you're an untrained beginner, however, you should always work with a rebirthing therapist.

BREATHER BEWARE

Breath awareness is not only habit-forming; it's very addictive. Once you start, there's no turning back. If you're not careful, you may even begin to feel really good all the time. You may even forget you were ever sick and tired and easily upset when you begin to experience more energy, aliveness, and joy. So breather, beware! If you're not ready to live the happy healthy life you were designed to live, then you may want to think twice before you take your first long, slow, full diaphragmatic breath.

ECODIET FUEL GROUP #3—FIRE

FUEL YOUR BODY THROUGH THE POWER OF THE SUN

The sun fuels all life on planet Earth. This fuel feeds the entire web of life. As I covered earlier, the first step is photosynthesis, in which the sun's radiant energy is turned into carbohydrate molecules by plants. We use these carbohydrates as another form of fuel for energy and as building blocks to build living cells.

Most believe the only way sunlight can fuel the human body is indirectly through plant foods, but let's explore another possible scenario. Imagine that your entire body is like a tree and the hairs on your body are the leaves.

Hairs, like leaves, act as receptors that absorb solar energy into their shafts, right through to the roots within our human tissues, and even deeper into our bodies. Just like a tree's roots need water, the leaves need sunlight. Just as our internal root system—the intestinal tract—needs water, that part of us that is exposed to the atmosphere—our skin—needs sunlight. Our body is of the solar system in which we live.

Unfortunately, most of us have lost our personal relationship with the sun. Historically, we've gone from worshipping it to shunning it. While every living thing upon our planet is dependent upon the light of the sun, we've been made to believe that it's our enemy. We've been taught that sunbathing and sungazing are dangerous practices that can destroy our retinas, age our skin, and cause cancer.

Current scientific research, however, exposes these myths. Let us now reconsider our on-again, off-again relationship with sunlight and open to an understanding of its importance in achieving a state of health and well-being.

EAT LIGHT

Vitamin D, the sunshine vitamin, is different from other vitamins in that it influences your entire body—receptors that respond to the vitamin have been found in almost every type of human cell, from your brain to your bones.

—Dr. Mark Sircus

Did you know that a lack of sufficient sunlight causes approximately one million deaths a year and that every living thing would eventually die without it? The human body, like all living things, receives more nourishment from the sun than most realize—yet we are sun-starved. Every cell in our body produces chemicals necessary for our life, and sunlight is the catalyst for the production of a vital chemical known as vitamin D. Recently, researchers from the Moore's Cancer Center at the University of California reported that if vitamin D3 levels among populations worldwide were increased, 600,000 cases of breast and colorectal cancers could be prevented each year. This includes nearly 150,000 cases of cancer that could be prevented in the United States alone. An inverse association between serum vitamin D and the risk of colorectal and breast cancers was also found.

Michael Holick, MD, an authority on vitamin D and the healing power of natural sunlight, says that sensible sun exposure during childhood not only maximizes the bone health of children, but it may even decrease their risk of chronic diseases in later life, including Type 1 diabetes, multiple sclerosis, rheumatoid arthritis, and common cancers.

Enjoying the sun is the best way to gain vitamin D. Nevertheless, if you're going to take a supplement, be sure to take vitamin D3. According to Australian researchers, the vitamin D that's added to milk and cereals (synthetic vitamin D2) suppresses the immune system—one more reason to shun milk.

Want to be healthier
SUNBATHE!

Several studies have shown that exposure to natural sunlight without sunscreen increases the number of white blood cells in the body, which plays a leading role in defending against invasions by bacteria and foreign organisms. Because of the increase in white blood cell activity after sunlight exposure, a person's ability to fight infections is greatly increased along with the body's ability to stop the reproduction of viruses. While it's important that we absorb the rays of the sun each day, like most anything else, sunbathing can be overdone. The sun must be treated with great respect. The skin must be properly conditioned to sunlight.

At higher latitudes (farther away from the equator), the angle of the sun's rays means that UV-B is available only for a few hours of the day. UV-B is the range of ultraviolet light that is needed for the production of vitamin D. In most of the United States, during the summer months, we need to be in the sun sometime between 10 am and 2 pm to stimulate vitamin D production. In the winter months, and in various places of the world where sunlight is at a minimal year-round, tanning beds or UV-B lamps can be very beneficial.

Add 5 to 10 minutes each day until you have a healthy, bronze tan. Keep in mind that the more skin exposure, the better.

So when it comes to feeding on sunlight, let it soak through your skin!

Want to protect your skin?
DRINK YOUR SUNSCREEN!

If you're a redhead or blonde with fair skin, you'll want to be especially considerate of the sun. But beware of sunscreens. Most sunscreen products cause more harm than good. Some sunscreen products contain toxic chemicals that, in penetrating through the skin, can actually increase the risk of disease. Toxic chemicals you may wish to avoid include: PABA, dioxybenzone, oxybenzone, titanium dioxide, and zinc oxide. Another major problem with sunscreen is that it blocks the skin's ability to produce vitamin D by more than 95%.

The answer to sun tolerance may be as simple as eating or drinking more fresh vegetables and berries—foods that are loaded with protective phytochemicals. Antioxidants protect our skin naturally. Nutrients such as polyphenols and vitamin C also offer protection from UVA radiation.

FOODS THAT PROTECT YOU

- Red, yellow, and orange fruits and veggies

  These contain carotenoid complexes, which reduce sunburn.

- Tart cherries and peppermint leaves

  These contain perilly alcohol, which stops cancer formation in human cells exposed to intense UV light.

- Leafy greens

  These contain lutein and zeaxanthin, which stops UV-induced cell proliferation.

- Green tea

  This contains antioxidant EGCGs, which block DNA damage in light-exposed human skin cells.

- Oranges, lemons, and limes
  These contain limonene, which is linked to a 34% reduction in skin cancer.

TRY ONE!

Try a cup of warm green tea in the morning or blend up a delectable fruit smoothie or juice a carotenoid-rich green drink *(see next page)*. The more you drink, the greater your protection.

Sunscreen Fruit Smoothie

1 large orange, peeled
12 strawberries, stemmed
1 banana, peeled
1 tablespoon green powder

Blend at high speed until
smooth.

Sunscreen Green Juice

8 stalks celery
4 kale or Swiss chard leaves
1 bunch parsley
1 handful spinach

Juice all of the above.

Want to become enlightened?
SUNGAZE!

Sungazing is a term broadly applied to an ancient practice of looking directly into the sun at sunrise or sunset. This practice takes place during the first or last 30 minutes of the day, when UV radiation is at its minimum. Look at the sun with a soft, relaxed focus for short periods of time initially, then gradually work up to longer amounts of time.

However, sungazing during a solar eclipse is not recommended. According to a technical paper published in the Bulletin of Mathematical Biophysics, thermal damage to the retina is possible when looking directly at a partial eclipse since only a little of the sun is exposed, and the pupil dilates to adapt to the low overall light level.

Daniel Reid, author of *The Tao of Detox* says:

> While the visible bands of light excite the retina's rods and cones to produce vision, the invisible ultraviolet band stimulates the adjacent epithelial cells, which transmit the stimulus as a powerful neural impulse through the optic nerve directly to the pituitary and pineal glands. Western medicine calls this newly discovered biosystem the "oculo-endocrine system."

There has not been much scientific evidence to substantiate the beneficial claims of sungazing, but there are numerous reports that suggest it is capable of providing the sungazer with a sense of physical, mental, emotional, and spiritual well-being. Some even report a decrease in irritability, anger, and frustration and an improvement in memory.

I can confirm those reports from my personal experience. I first began sungazing when I lived on the beach in Costa Rica. I would gaze at the sun as it rose over the ocean at dawn. It gave me a feeling of peaceful contentment that I had never really felt before. I could almost understand what sun worship was about in those ancient days. I wrote some of my greatest poetry during that time.

However, I was also eating a diet of almost exclusively fruit. I would pick avocados and bananas, mangoes, coconuts, and pineapples from the grounds where we lived. I don't think it would have even entered my mind to sungaze if I hadn't already been eating a diet of solar-charged, raw plant foods. I believe that plant foods prepare us for the direct experience of a relationship with the sun.

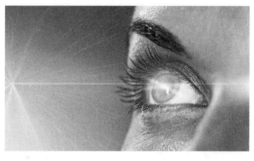

Sungazing is often practiced with bare feet in direct contact with the earth. You begin by looking directly at the rising sun for ten seconds then adding an additional ten seconds to the total sungazing time each consecutive day until you are looking at the sun for up to 45 minutes.

Some sungazers have experienced the feeling of hunger dissipate after six months, and after ten months some have claimed that they no longer feel the need to eat! It is alleged that after 45 minutes of sungazing, one would be full of light energy, just like a solar-charged battery. If these claims hold true, the implications could be staggering.

Want a slim trim body?

EAT LIGHT!

If you live in areas of the world that experience dark and cold seasons, you're probably familiar with seasonal affective disorder (SAD). SAD is a disorder that occurs when lack of sunlight causes a drop in the level of the neurotransmitter serotonin in the brain. This drop results in mood changes such as depression. Not only can a drop in serotonin levels affect your mood, it may also affect other things such as your appetite and your feelings of hunger and satiation.

Hunger is largely controlled by a part of your brain called the hypothalamus. The hypothalamus works with serotonin to relieve feelings of hunger. As the body reaches its needed caloric intake, serotonin is released, causing a feeling of fullness. With a lack of sunlight, a drop in serotonin levels can result in the feeling of fullness being delayed. This can cause a greater calorie intake during times when sunlight is not as prevalent.

Another way that sunlight may play a role in the regulation of appetite has to do with Brobeck's theory of heat production. This theory states that as body temperature drops, you feel hungrier. As body temperature rises, you feel less hungry. This can result in greater caloric consumption during times of the year with less sunlight.

Sungazing may also affect your appetite—at any time of year. I've sun-gazed at various times over last 15 to 20 years, usually for about 10 minutes once or twice a day. During those times, I found that I wasn't that hungry. But the lack of hunger felt more like it was coming from the peaceful contentment I felt. It may have been more an effect on the emotional addictions around eating.

Whatever the reason or method, whether through sunbathing or sungazing, sunlight is nature's greatest appetite suppressor. So use the light of the sun to slim down!

Want to oxygenate your blood?
BECOME A LIGHT ABSORBER!

Red blood cells contain hemoglobin, a ring-shaped molecule much like chlorophyll, the light-processing molecule in plants. The main difference is that the coordinating atom in hemoglobin is iron, and in chlorophyll it is magnesium. It is not so surprising then, to find out that hemoglobin is also a light-processing molecule. In fact, there is now a new technology for monitoring hemoglobin by measuring light absorption.

It is common knowledge that blood containing high levels of oxygen is a bright red color. The spent blood that has delivered its load of oxygen to the cells has a deep bluish tinge. This color change is another indication that hemoglobin absorbs light—in different ranges, depending on the level of oxygenation.

In The Hygienic System (1934), Herbert Shelton, a strong advocate of fasting and sunbathing, wrote, "Sunlight dominates the chemistry of the blood. People who do not get sunlight do not have the same richness and redness of blood as do those who secure plenty of sunlight."

So, if you can, be a light absorber—through the eyes, the skin, and the blood. Sunlight directly energizes the blood for its tasks of oxygenation and alkalization.

SUNBATHER BEWARE

Like breath awareness, gazing, and bathing in light is very addictive. It can even be intoxicating. Once you start soaking in the rays of the sun, there's no stopping. If you are not careful, you may begin to feel happy and energized. You may find it opens you up to a deeper relationship to those you love. You may find that you've gone down a size or two. So beware! If you're not ready to live in a healthy, slim, bronzed body then you may want to think twice before soaking in the light of the sun!

ECODIET FUEL GROUP #4—WATER
FUEL YOUR BODY THROUGH THE POWER OF WATER

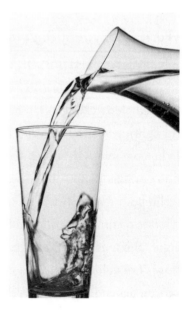

Water is truly the gift of life; without it, there would be no life in the physical world. Every life form that exists on Earth is conceived in and born out of water. Even the human body takes form in a water sac held within our mother's womb. Once the nine-month gestation period is complete, the water breaks and we are born, within billions of water molecules.

In terms of the number of molecules, your body actually consists of over 99% water molecules!

—Dr. Gerald Pollack

Within living systems, everything happens in water. By weight,

- your muscles consist of 75% water,
- your brain consists of 90% water,
- your bones consist of 22% water, and
- your blood consists of 83% water.

And, remember, water by weight is 90% oxygen so if you are dehydrated, your body is going to be low in oxygen, which makes your internal environment vulnerable to microbial invasions.

SUFFERING FROM AN INTERNAL DROUGHT?

While a lack of water supply in the human body is called dehydration, it could also be called an internal drought. Internal droughts take place whenever your water supply is low—much like the earth without rainfall. An insufficient water supply stresses the body and our cells wilt, like a plant in dry soil.

We also need a greater flow of water when there are toxins stored in the body. The more toxins and acid wastes, the greater the need for water to dilute them and flush them through.

Water regulates every function in the body and whenever there is an insufficient water supply, everything suffers. Thus, it is easy to imagine how dehydration might just play a significant part in disease and death.

Dehydration causes the blood to separate into both watery and thicker, stickier fractions. Consequently, more energy is required to pump the blood into the farther reaches of the body.

As the rate of flow is reduced, greater pressures are exerted to keep the blood moving. Movement of nutrients and wastes between blood vessels and cells is compromised. With less efficient removal of acid wastes and poor oxygenation in an already congested bloodstream, cells begin to either bloat or wilt, and their functions decline.

Stagnation begins to occur in weaker areas of the body, perhaps where the stickier blood clumps around miniscule obstructions in blood vessels or openings. Depending on where the internal drought has settled, the initial indicators are different in different people.

THE NEW SCIENCE OF STRUCTURED WATER

We must also consider the qualities of the waters, for as they differ from one another in taste and weight, so also do they differ much in their qualities.

—Hippocrates

In pristine nature, water is perfectly structured. In constant, dynamic movement, water literally has the ability to purify itself. Water in a mountain stream passes over and around stones and other obstacles—parting and swirling around them on either side, which purifies and highly charges the water. The flows and counter flows create vortexes, which break up large, low-energy molecular clusters into smaller, high-energy clusters. This type of dynamic movement also lowers the surface tension of water and creates beneficial structuring. This kind of water is instantaneously useable at the cellular level.

Dr. Mu Shik Jhon, author of *The Water Puzzle and the Hexagonal Key,* found that water molecules near abnormal cells were disorderly and more highly mutable than those near the normal cells. He reported, "structured water in cells play the role in maintaining normal condition of the cells and if, for some reason, the structure of water is damaged, cancer or diabetes arises."

The natural, dynamic flow of structured water has the ability to isolate and dissolved toxins. It energetically neutralizes toxins (including free radicals) and energetically enhances nutrients. Toxins held within the matrix of this water move through the body and are eliminated without causing damage. As long as the water is moving, toxic pollutants cannot destroy the structure. In a world of increasingly contaminated water, this is something powerful to understand.

In nature, there are other factors involved in the structuring of water—for instance, the sun. According to Gerald Pollack, PhD, a professor of bioengineering at the University of Washington, radiant energy structures water. It structures the water in a mountain stream, and it structures the water in your body, especially when you sunbathe or sungaze.

Finally, walking on the earth sustains the molecular structure of water in your body. When you walk barefoot on the earth, you absorb electrons from the negatively charged earth through the soles of your feet, which assists in alkalizing the waters of your body…

just be sure to choose a safe place to walk, in an area that hasn't been chemically treated.

If you drink water that has been naturally structured you may notice:

- a smoother, mellower flavor;
- a sense of expansiveness in the mouth;
- an immediate sense of mental clarity, physical energy, and emotional ease;
- and a desire to drink more!

Want to prevent inflammation in your body?
FILTER YOUR TAP WATER!

Most tap water contains a stew of chemicals, from nitrates in farming regions, to pharmaceutical drugs, radioactive particles, and industrial toxins. It is treated with chlorine and fluorides. It then flows through pipes under pressure, which breaks down the natural structure of water.

According to the Environmental Working Group, there have been at least 315 pollutants found in America's tap water since 2004, and over half of these pollutants are unregulated and can legally exist in any amount. Many of these chemicals are synthetic petrochemical derivatives.

Using products with petrochemicals causes inflammation in the body.
This type of inflammation is what causes many types of cancer.

–Deepak Chopra, M.D.

When you don't drink enough water, and the water you drink is polluted, not only do the cells wilt, they can also become raw and inflamed. Over time, pollutants tend to collect in areas of drought, where congestion obstructs the removal of toxins. Like food scraps on dishes instead of being rinsed off, they become dried on and hardened; the pollutants stay on as biological irritants.

One of the most common contaminants in our water is fluoride. Activist Jeff Green says, "fluoride is used in the ceramics business to make ceramics more porous. Well, it does exactly the same thing to your bones." The government ordered to have fluoride added to the water in order to reduce cavities and tooth decay, in other words for the purposes of medication. Unfortunately, there are numerous hazards to this chemical; for example, studies show that babies exposed to fluoride are at high risk of developing dental fluorosis—a permanent tooth defect caused by fluoride damaging the cells which form the teeth. In fact, 97% of Western Europe has chosen fluoride-free water.

John Yiamouyiannis, Ph.D., author of *Fluoride The Aging Factor,* remonstrates: "We would not purposely add arsenic to the water supply. And we would not purposely add lead. But we do add fluoride. The fact is that fluoride is more toxic than lead and just slightly less toxic than arsenic."

While fluoride is dangerous enough, the type of fluoride added to municipal water systems is not pharmaceutical grade but an industrial waste product that also contains heavy metals (including lead and arsenic), radioactive products, and other contaminants from the phosphate fertilizer industry.

In 1992, Robert Carton, Ph.D., a former EPA scientist, declared, "Fluoridation is the greatest scientific fraud of this century, if not of all time!"

In 1998, the union representing fifteen hundred scientists, lawyers, engineers and other professional employees of the Environmental Protection Agency took a stand opposing the fluoridation of drinking water supplies and tried to sue its own agency for ignoring the important data on the dangers of fluoridation. It was unsuccessful.

As you can see, finding the right kind of water to drink has become a real issue.

Want to be healthier?
DON'T TREAT THIRST WITH MEDICATION!

It's a fact, nothing destroys life quicker than a lack of water—whether in our internal environment, or in the world we live in. It's also a fact that people with the worst health generally drink the least amount of water, and instead drink the most dehydrating drinks, such as caffeinated and alcoholic beverages.

F. Batmanghelidj, MD, author of *Your Body's Many Cries for Water*, found in his years of research that Unintentional Chronic Dehydration (UCD) contributes to and even produces disabilities and degenerative diseases, such as cancer, Type 2 diabetes, heart disease, depression, obesity, addictions, and others. He believes that with the right quality and quantity of water, you can "cure the sick."

He says, "I have used water to cure people who were suffering from "incurable" diseases. I have cured people who suffered for 10 years, 20 years, even 30 years from painful conditions produced by dehydration. In short, you're not sick; you're thirsty. Do not treat thirst with medication!"

To think that so much suffering can be prevented and treated simply by increasing water intake on a regular basis is astonishing, isn't it?

In the initial stages of dehydration, the body releases stress hormones. In chronic dehydration, the body is mobilized in a continuous state of "fight or flight," as if you are living in a dangerous world. And you are!

An internal drought affects every part of the internal environment. Whether drought stress triggers high blood pressure, headaches, asthma or obesity is a matter of the constitutional weaknesses and trauma-holding patterns of each person. Drink more water and watch your internal dessert bloom!

But it is not all about quantity. The structural quality (meaning its ionic composition) of water also matters. Dr. Pollack tells us, "the water inside your cells is absolutely critical for your health. If you have a particular pathology of an organ, it's not only the proteins inside that organ that are not working, but also the water inside that organ. That near-protein water is not ordered in the way it should be."

We have been taught to believe that water has three phases—solid (ice), liquid (water), and gas (water vapor). Pollack posits a fourth phase of water—a liquid crystalline phase that we call structured water. He is convinced that the water in the cells is mainly this kind of ordered water.

Much of the water in the universe may be like a liquid crystal.

—Gerald Pollack

Want a slim, trim body?
YOU'RE NOT HUNGRY—YOU'RE THIRSTY!

Water is nature's greatest weight-loss secret. Dr. Batmanghelidj has come to the conclusion that gaining weight is one of the body's adaptive responses to chronic dehydration.

Dr. Howard Flaks, an obesity specialist in Beverly Hills, agrees:

> By not drinking enough water, many people incur excess body fat, poor muscle tone and size, decreased digestive efficiency and organ function, increased toxicity in the body, joint and muscle soreness and water retention.

Dr. Batmanghelidj's studies have shown that, for most people, the thirst mechanism is so weak that it is often mistaken for hunger.

He says:

You are not hungry—you are thirsty!

The great news is that for most people one glass of water will shut down hunger pangs. Not only does water suppress the appetite, causing you to eat fewer calories, it also helps the body metabolize stored fat.

This is because the kidneys aren't able to function properly without adequate amounts of water and when they don't work to capacity, some of their load is dumped onto the liver. One of the liver's primary functions is to metabolize stored fat into usable energy for the body. Thus, if the liver is forced to do some of the kidney's work, it can't operate at full throttle. As a result, it metabolizes less fat. Even mild dehydration will slow down one's metabolism.

If you want to look good, keep in mind that water helps to maintain proper muscle tone by giving muscles their natural ability to contract. Drinking plenty of water also helps to prevent the sagging skin that usually follows weight loss. Shrinking cells are buoyed by water, which plumps the skin and leaves it clear, healthy, and resilient.

For faster rehydration, drink cool (59°–72°) water. To curb your appetite, drink warmer water. Warmer water doesn't leave the stomach as quickly, so a sensation of fullness may linger.

Want to prevent aging?
DRINK WATER!

Dehydration is one of the greatest triggers of free radicals in the body. Water is the greatest free radical remover. Free radicals are a prime cause of rapid aging, as they damage the cell's architecture.

While the average adult's body is around 75% water, as we age, it can dip as low as 65% for men and 52% for women. Then, at the brink of death, this can drop another 10%. Dehydration and its correlation with life and death are synonymous throughout nature. Think of plants and leaves that are dead or dying. They dry up and become brittle and fragile just before they are declared dead. Or, consider a grape and how it becomes a raisin!

Most people literally shrink and wither as they age (wrinkles, loss of height, and muscle mass) due to dehydration.

Again, the quality of water is also crucial. There may be such a thing as "dead" water, meaning that it has lost its ionic charge.

> *When we die, all of the structure is lost. Being alive is really the same perhaps as saying that we're filled with this kind of water.*
>
> —Gerald Pollack, PhD

Searching for peak performance?
CHARGE YOUR WATER BATTERIES!

Peak performance is dependent on an adequate water supply. One example illustrates this perfectly: two European mountain-climbing teams were competing. One team was in better physical condition than the other team, but was unable to win. That team started to carefully study the other team's every move. They noticed that after so many minutes of climbing, each team member drank water. Copying this water-drinking habit resulted in victory. No longer were they lacking the vital nutrient needed. Optimum water consumption was the key.

You can see from this example that drinking water gave the climbers energy. You may know that every cell in your body has a self-replicating power plant called the mitochondrion. This power plant breaks down glucose for energy through aerobic respiration—that is, through oxygen. However, did you know that in addition to the mitochondrial power plants, there are water batteries at every microscopic surface in the body?

Dr. Pollack and his colleagues found that water molecules are structured in an orderly fashion at the surfaces of a cell membrane. At these surfaces, there's a separation of charge in the water. Negative charges collect closest to the surface, in what is called an exclusion zone, and positive charges collect just beyond that zone. It is like a battery!

Dr. Pollack explains "You have to charge these batteries and the question is: how are these batteries charged? It comes from incident radiant energy—light, heat, and ultraviolet radiation. It is the energy that is coming in from outside that creates this potential energy of order and charge separation. This potential energy fills your cells." If you think about it, the energy that charges these batteries ultimately comes from the sun.

It is easy to imagine, then, that when a person is dehydrated, the movement of fluids in the body becomes sluggish, and the liquid structure begins to break down. The water batteries run down and you, in turn, feel sluggish, like a car chugging up a hill.

This new understanding of microscopic "water batteries" within us may spark future research in the generation of electrical power from sunlight and water!

TIPS FOR STAYING HYDRATED

- Start each day with a large glass of structured water—even before you brush your teeth. Drinking structured water first thing in the morning replaces the fluids lost overnight and gets your hydration efforts off to a great start. If you wish, add the juice of one lemon.

- Eat two or three servings of raw fruits and vegetables at every meal, or drink freshly-prepared juices. They are brimming with structured water and include the alkaline mineral electrolytes that recharge the body.

- Eliminate toxic, acid-forming foods. They result in a lowering of your body's water table, depleting your electrolytes. Then, the body struggles to dilute and eliminate acid wastes.

- Avoid plastic bottles whenever possible. If you work outside of the home, fill a glass quart bottle with structured water to take with you in the car, or keep it with you and refill it during the workday.

- If you know that you get really busy through the day and forget to drink water, establish regular water breaks. Tailor your drinking to meet your needs. For instance, drink extra water in the morning. Or if you work out, or haven't included enough fruits and vegetables during the day, drink extra water an hour before bedtime.

FUEL GRADES OF WATER

We tend to take water for granted. We don't even notice its clear, mirror-like quality, or appreciate the way it sparkles in the light. Unless the water is contaminated, the taste is like the taste of our own spit—easy to disregard. Yet water and the quality of water is so important to our life.

REGULAR FUEL

While tap water may appear to be clean, it is usually "dirty fuel." This is because of the chemicals that leach into the environment as part of our petrochemical lifestyle, and the chemicals that are added at the drinking water treatment plant—things like chlorides and fluorides, and the hazardous wastes that come along with fluoridation.

The first step in improving the quality of your tap water is filtration. Basic filtration involves removal of small particulate matter and activated carbon filtration to remove chlorine and some volatile organic compounds (VOCs). Beyond that, the home filter that works best for you will depend on the specific problems that are found in tap water in your area.

A good place to start your research is with the Environmental Working Group website: *http://www.ewg.org/tap-water/getawaterfilter*. Here you can enter your zip code, or the name of your water company, and get your local test results. Then you can find out which filters would work best for you.

A whole house filter is the best way to go, if possible. You "drink" water not only through your mouth, but also through your skin.

MIDGRADE FUEL

So now you have filtered water that is reasonably pure. The problem is that in moving through the underground pipes of the city and even through the filtration system, the water that comes out of your faucet has lost its charge and natural structure. What you need is a way to restructure the water, to bring it back to vibrant life.

There are water units that will restructure the water. These water units generally use flow forms to revitalize the water through spiraling vortexes of movement. Vortexing erases the memory of impurities and simultaneously creates a molecular structure that protects the body from any remaining impurities. There are many different water-structuring machines coming onto the market now.

You can install a whole house unit in your home and use a portable unit while traveling or at the office. Structured water is important for drinking, but also for showering, bathing, and watering the garden. The garden plants will show you their appreciation, too. The unit I use and the one I most highly recommend can be found in the resource section.

PREMIUM FUEL

Because your body is slightly alkaline by design, the water you drink should also be slightly alkaline. When you drink alkaline water (up to pH 8.5), it readily escorts oxygen into your cells and tissues and ushers out acids and toxic wastes. There are countertop machines on the market that ionize and alkalize water. While the strong electric current used to produce ionized, alkaline water may not create the same kind of structuring that the gentler, natural movement of vortexing produces, it does create a type of structured water with benefits in resolving some of our modern diseases.

For short-term cleansing or disease conditions such as cancer or diabetes, a strongly alkaline water of pH 9.5 can be highly beneficial. A number of my friends and acquaintances have reversed various health challenges by using ionized, alkaline water, so I'm a strong advocate. I've seen what it can do.

THE POWER OF COLONIC HYDROTHERAPY

Another way to prepare your body for full hydration is to directly flush accumulated toxic waste from your colon with lots and lots of water. When the colon is clean and healthy, it does not provide a stagnant environment conducive to the onset of disease. Instead, it is able to fully utilize the water you drink to draw out wastes.

In 1913, the subject of alimentary toxemia was discussed in London before the Royal Society of Medicine by 57 leading physicians of Great Britain. Among the speakers were eminent surgeons, physicians and specialists in various branches of medicine. A report of the proceedings notes that many chronic diseases are principally caused by an infection of the gastrointestinal tract. It should be understood that these findings were not mere theories, but the results of demonstrations in actual practice by some of the most eminent physicians of the time.

Dr. Diana Schwarzbein, MD, author of *The Schwarzbein Principle* says, "It has been estimated that 70 to 80% of the cells of the immune system are located in the digestive tract. Therefore, if you are already experiencing any health symptoms, conditions or have a degenerative disease of aging, you have a problem with your digestive tract."

Therefore, keeping our colon clean and the beneficial micro-populations of your digestive system happy and healthy is the foundation of a strong immune system.

Dr. Bernard Jensen, DC, ND, PhD, one of the world's leading authorities on colon health says, "It is ironic that in spite of our modern external sanitation, we give precious little thought to taking care of our personal internal sanitation…We must learn to take proper care of our inner environment so that we can avoid disease and encourage health."

In essence, the colon is the sewage system of our body, but by neglect and abuse it can become a backed-up, toxic cesspool. Therefore, cleansing the colon with colon hydrotherapy is vitally important.

Colon hydrotherapy, also known as a colonic, flushes the colon with gallons of warm filtered water. You can either go to a professional colon hydrotherapist or you can do it yourself in the privacy of your home by using a home colonic board.

The cost of a professional colonic treatment is about $60 per session. You change into a gown and lie on a padded table so that the colon hydrotherapist can insert a sterile, double-lumen tube gently into the anus. The colon is then gently flushed with repeated doses of warmed water, which loosens waste stuck in the colon and filters it out through the tube system.

The cost of a home colonic board (also called a colema board) is around $300. Setting up a colonic irrigation unit at home will save you hundreds of dollars in the long run. After your fifth session, you will have paid for your board while using it for many years thereafter. It's a very wise investment indeed.

When giving yourself (or anyone else) a colonic or enema, be sure to use the highest quality of water possible—pure, structured water with some prayer or appropriate positive thoughts added, perhaps.

Colon hydrotherapy is a wonderful way to assist your body in any cleansing program. Dr. Jensen recommended at least two to three colonic irrigations per week during his cleansing programs. Dr. Richard Anderson, author of *Cleanse and Purify Thyself*, also recommends colonics or enemas during his cleansing programs.

Any time you have a reaction to cleansing—headache, low energy, and grumpiness, whatever it may be—washing the toxins out of your colon is the answer. You could even have cleansing effects by moving into the *EcoDiet* program more quickly than your body can easily adjust.

The answer? Colon hydrotherapy!

USE YOUR MIND AND EMOTIONS TO STRUCTURE YOUR INTERNAL WATERS

Whether mental, emotional, electromagnetic, chemical, or physical, unresolved stresses create a kind of stasis that keeps the environment of the body in a drought-like condition. Unresolved stress is part of the process through which cellular communication becomes fragmented. The tension of an emotional holding pattern has a negative effect on all of your bodily functions.

When you suppress signals of underlying emotional distress, the mind becomes less receptive and aware of other signals, like the signals of thirst that your body naturally gives you. You may open the refrigerator with the vague idea that you are hungry, when you are actually thirsty. Confused responses become entangled with confused signals of thirst (headaches, coughing, fuzzy thinking, little aches and pains). You may believe you are not thirsty only because cellular communication has broken down.

While water is one of the most common substances on Earth, we spend little time thinking about this mysterious liquid that keeps us alive. But the world is starting to open its eyes to the wonders of this miracle substance—its mysteries, its ancient significance, and its ability to structure consciousness and remember anything that comes into contact with it.

Water's molecular bonding structures are formed by everything that surrounds it, including human thoughts and emotions. For instance, the latest findings surrounding consciousness and water show that a simple blessing can have positive effects on the structure of water.

Dr. Masaru Emoto, researcher and author of *Hidden Messages in Water* has demonstrated how our thoughts and emotions impact our health. He found that the structure of water is influenced for better or worse when exposed to different types of music, spoken words, written words, videos, and pictures.

By freezing water, then photographing the thawing water crystals, Dr. Emoto discovered crystalline structures in water that reveal images of thoughts and emotions. He found that water from clear springs and water that has been exposed to loving words shows brilliant, complex, and colorful snowflake patterns. In contrast, polluted water, or water exposed to negative thoughts, forms incomplete, asymmetrical patterns with dull colors.

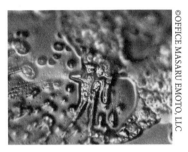
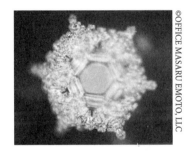

YOU MAKE ME SICK   LOVE AND GRATITUDE

His research has created a new awareness of how our thoughts can positively impact the earth and our personal health.

Cancer specialist Dr. Leonard Coldwell concedes that while you may follow a protocol for curing cancer, "the main cause of cancer is mental and emotional stress…Therefore I would know that I have to uncover and eliminate the root cause of my personal health challenge to be able to get rid of the symptoms and physical malfunction." Of course, cancer is just one example. Other degenerative diseases can have mental and emotional roots, as well.

Thus, considering that our bodies are made up of mostly water, maybe we had better think twice before entertaining another negative thought.

So think good thoughts and drink up! You'll be glad you did!

WATER HYDRATOR BEWARE

Hydrating your body with lots of structured water every day is very addictive. Like breath awareness, sunbathing, and eating plant foods, once you start hydrating your body the way nature intended, there is no turning back. If you are not careful, you may become so hydrated that all of your health problems vanish. You may even discover that you feel really good all the time. So beware! If you're not ready to live in a healthy, hydrated body, you may want to think twice before drinking lots of structured water!

CONCLUSION

ECODIET
THE ECOTARIAN VISION

A diet is not intended to be something you go "on" one day then "off" the next. It's a lifestyle—a habitual way of eating that reflects your interconnectedness to the web of life.

Perhaps you are among those of us who are sensing that change is in the air. The earth is shifting; we are shifting. A new world is upon us.

While I was meditating one day, I asked God what my mission was at this critical time on our planet. That's when I heard my inner voice say that my purpose at this time was to assist people in getting their physical bodies ready for the change that is occurring on planet Earth. While I wasn't fully sure what that meant at the time, I now know more. This mission has been my underlying purpose in writing *EcoDiet* and living the ecotarian lifestyle.

To most of us, it appears that we are separate from God or our living earth, but we are not. Our physical bodies are made up of the same elemental substances as the earth. How we thrive and how we die is one and the same. We have polluted our earth—our very habitat. We have polluted our bodies—our spirit's habitat.

But, there is another way. We hold the keys of transformation for a return to our original nature, which will simultaneously assist the earth in doing the same; this is our interconnected mission—the vision held within the heart of an *ecotarian*.

In Part I, I introduced the concept of eating according to our natural design. When we choose an acidic diet of animal products and processed, chemicalized foods, we create a type of internal acid rain, similar to the acid rain that is slowly but surely destroying our planet. On the other hand, when we consume foods that we were anatomically designed to eat, we create a thriving alkaline environment, replete with oxygen and free from sickness and disease.

The key is our body's pH. When we choose an alkalizing diet of organic, fresh fruits and greens, along with a small amount of nuts and seeds, our internal environment thrives!

We have learned that our health is directly connected to the health of the earth, each held within a complex and delicate web of existence. The ways in which our body thrives or dies are strikingly similar to the ways in which the earth thrives or dies. If the physicians and scientists of our time could connect these ecological dots, medicine as we know it would come to an end.

We've seen how our simultaneous belief in Pasteur's germ theory and denial of Antoine Béchamp's internal terrain theory has created a culture (along with mega-industries) that is devoted to conquering an enemy (germs) that continues to demonstrate its pleomorphic (shape and size-shifting) invincibility.

I've offered a foundational cause of our problems in the erroneous perspectives that arise from the illusion of separation. I've also put forth my own theory of internal acid rain as an explanation for the progression of disease.

Finally, you now have some simple in-home tests—for candida and pH—to gauge the general condition of your internal environment.

In Part II, we gained a critical awareness of what is happening to our food supply, and how it is affecting humanity and all living creatures around the globe.

Dietary devolution is plummeting to new lows as pesticides contaminate our foods and bodies, and drugs and chemicals replace natural, living foods—the foods that sustain human life. The corruption of our food supply, including the widespread proliferation of genetically modified foods (GMOs), which can affect our DNA structure thereby aiding in a decreased immunity, is not only destroying our body's ecological balance, it is destroying the ecological balance of our planet.

So, I invite you to join me in reversing the disastrous trends afflicting us now, and become part of the *Ecotarian Revolution.* Make a commitment to restore the health of your body, even if it means turning away from the messages of mainstream agriculture, food purveyors, and medical establishments. In saving ourselves, we are also playing a huge part in saving the billions of other life forms around us, and our Earth.

The natural, living foods of the earth have their own delicious flavors, but these flavors are greatly reduced by conventional farming methods and long periods of storage and travel. In place of natural flavors, we most often reach for the enticing, habit-forming flavors of salt, oil, and sugar.

By sounding the alarm—an S-O-S—on **S**alt, **O**il and **S**ugar, the three primary offenders that corrupt our taste buds and keep food cravings and addictions in place, we take the first steps toward becoming an ecotarian. Replacing the wrong kinds of salt, oil, and sugar with better choices improves every meal we eat.

Then, we begin to truly nourish and sustain the body with living foods, and shift our pH for greater alkalinity and oxygenation.

In Part III, I laid out a simple program for you to follow and develop an ecotarian lifestyle. When you practice natural feeding from the *four fuel groups*—taking time to breathe mindfully, connect with the sun, drink high-energy water throughout the day, and eat the plant foods of the earth—you will finally come to know, as I have, what it truly means to be fully alive and to thrive.

In *EcoDiet*, I have laid out three grades of fuel: *regular* beginner vegetarian fare, *midgrade* intermediate or advanced vegan fare, and *premium* master ecotarian fare. Start by enjoying any one of the delicious, alkalizing recipes in this book. However, if you are seriously ill, I highly recommend going straight to the *master ecotarian plan* under the care and guidance of a natural health professional. Otherwise, you may want to allow your body to adjust to your new ways by taking one step at a time.

The EcoDiet, which should be so natural and easy, is actually a radical departure from the lifestyles of most modern Americans. We've moved away from Hippocrates' (the founder of modern medicine) precept of *making food your medicine and medicine your food*. We no longer understand what it means to *sit at nature's table*, or have a true understanding of food—its purpose and its power. Commercial infrastructures have largely replaced our natural way of being. Our highways are literally lined with fast-"food" restaurants fashionably equipped with drive-thru windows offering quick and inexpensive hunger fixes—incredibly tempting when our bodies are calling for fuel and we are short on time. Like me, the question you have to ask yourself before consuming this fast food is: *What is the cost to the internal environment of my body and to the planet—today, tomorrow, and in the years ahead—in making this decision?*

With time, I finally learned to just say "NO!" to processed foods that acidify me and create a toxic internal environment conducive to germs, sickness, and disease. I also learned to say "YES!" to foods that alkalize me and create a pristine internal environment conducive to health—physical, mental, emotion, and spiritual well-being.

While it took a little time and lots of discipline, my body no longer craves the foods that destroy my health; now my body craves foods that support the sustainability of my internal environment. The challenge facing us now is that time has nearly run out.

With the depletion of natural resources and the levels of pollution alone, we no longer have the luxury that I had, to *slowly* adopt the principles set forth in EcoDiet and for living the ecotarian lifestyle; Mother Earth will not be able to sustain the human race as long as we continue to destroy her. Can you imagine what would be possible if we would get busy *now* and embrace the critical changes necessary for reducing our footprint and ensuring health and life for ourselves and all other life forms while encouraging others to do the same? The possibilities are wonderful and limitless for sure.

It may not be easy for some of you to adopt the EcoDiet. It is human nature, typically, to wait until we are faced with our own mortality by way of disease before taking imperative steps. However, if you follow the guidelines in this book, and exercise your free will in this new direction you will persevere, trust me.

I know, firsthand, what it takes to say "NO!" to old food habits and cravings. It takes discipline as I mentioned before, but it also takes clarity and vision—clarity about how you want to feel and operate within this web of life, and a vision of some possible outcomes as a result of you taking these steps. The discipline will only be necessary for a short time, until your body, mind, and emotions can break its addictions. Then, before you know it, you will be on your way to living a new and vibrant life with numerous unexpected gifts.

The sky is the limit when you feel happy and energized in life; your moods, your creativity, and your desire and ability to help others will all improve and increase. What is possible for you in this place is exponential.

Believe me when I tell you that prior to becoming sick I was walking in similar shoes as many of you. Now, I live my life to its fullest, guided by spirit with an unexplainable joy for life, which now has a depth that I never dreamed was possible.

Here is the one secret that everyone who has succeeded in adopting the EcoDiet knows: *When you say "YES!" to life and living foods, life says "YES!" to you.*

This means, when you feed your body the foods your body was designed to eat (fruits and vegetables, along with a few nuts, and seeds), after about ninety days those are the only foods you will crave! It's all about breaking old habits. Even in the moments when you have a "snack attack" brought on by a drop in blood sugar or a stressful moment, you just might find yourself reaching for an organic banana, or a raw, dehydrated flaxseed cracker and some delicious sweet Muscadine grapes, rather than a Coke and a bag of Doritos, or a Snickers Bar.

Even though I've written more about plant foods from the earth as fuel than the other three fuel groups—sun, water, and air—this does not mean that "earth" foods are the most important "fuel" group. Sunlight, air, and water are just as essential to life as foods from the earth! In fact one cannot exist without the other. I now know that the sunlight, fresh air, and living water have a power to alkalize and revitalize your internal environment beyond most scientific comprehension. These three elements provide amazing energy to every single cell of our body, while providing boundless benefits to our mind, emotions, and spirit. So, make sure to "eat" from nature's dynamic *four fuel groups* every day!

In writing this book, I have practiced what I preach—searching, studying, experimenting, and finally choosing the best possible information to share with you. Like they have for me, the sun will sustain you, pure water will hydrate you, and the recipes that I have shared with you will alkalize you.

However, in my journey, the element of air through the power of deep, conscious breathing has been, perhaps, the most powerful transformational tool of all. (Make sure to review and practice the breathing exercises that I go into detail starting on page 212.) Most people are surprised about how different and good they feel when they practice conscious breathing every day throughout the day. In my estimation, this is one of the most important and mighty health "foods" of all!

This book and the guidelines and program set forth as the EcoDiet are a snapshot in time. My understanding of things continues to evolve day by day, as will yours. So rather than taking my word for it, I invite you to try it out and see for yourself.

By making the choice to follow the principles of the EcoDiet and eating in harmony with your body's natural design, you are, in essence, transitioning into an ecotarian lifestyle, while becoming a part of a major shift that will revolutionize our world.

This is why I'm calling this movement the *Ecotarian Revolution*!

Ecotarian Revolution—A way of living that supports
the sustainability of our body and planet!

THE *ECOTARIAN REVOLUTION*: A PARADIGM SHIFT

When I shared with you the story of how I almost died, I gave you a key that is very close to my heart: *There is only one problem, ever: the illusion of separation.* Sadly, most of us hold the belief, consciously or unconsciously, that we are somehow separate from God, nature, the earth, and everyone that appears to be outside of us. It's when we hold this belief in separation that we become self-centered and self-serving. Breaking the spell of this belief is the first step in transforming ourselves and our planet back into our original designs, and it's a step that we all must ultimately take.

If we continue to live in the illusion of separation, we will continue to make choices (individually and collectively) that lead us down the path of devolution toward disease and death, and eventual extinction.

My hope is that in recognizing and embracing natural feeding, and restoring the health and vibrancy of your internal environment, you will grasp a powerful means to end the various illusions of separation that may be at play in your own life.

Simply remember the words of Albert Einstein,

A human being is a part of the whole, called by us "Universe," a part limited
in time and space. He experiences himself, his thoughts and feelings as
somethingseparated from the rest—a kind of optical delusion of his consciousness.
This delusion is a kind of prison for us, restricting us to our personal desires
and to affection for a few persons nearest to us. Our task must be to free ourselves
from this prison by widening our circle of compassion to embrace all living
creatures and the whole of nature in its beauty.

Ultimately, the *Ecotarian Revolution* is not about becoming a vegetarian, vegan, or fruitarian. It is about an ecotarian lifestyle that supports the sustainability of our body and the planet. It is about the realization of our bodies as living ecosystems and the willingness to take our true place within the larger ecosystems of the earth.

It is about a paradigm shift. It is about being the change we want to see in the world! Just as we have a pH scale, we also have a paradigm scale.

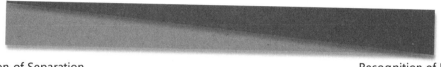

Illusion of Separation   Recognition of Unity

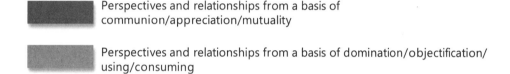

Perspectives and relationships from a basis of communion/appreciation/mutuality

Perspectives and relationships from a basis of domination/objectification/using/consuming

The Paradigm Scale

A move toward the right on the pH scale is the physical equivalent to a move toward the right on the paradigm scale of human consciousness. Eating the flesh of animals and other unnatural foods keeps us locked into the acidic end of the scale—aggressive, fearful, and domineering—while eating the "flesh" of fruit will unlock the essence of our alkaline nature—loving, compassionate, and cooperative.

With time, an EcoDiet will clean out the toxic, acidic wastes that veil your true nature, helping you to release old patterns of thoughts and emotions that no longer serve your highest and best. Just as releasing the acidic wastes in the body takes time, a paradigm shift is also accompanied by toxic emotional patterns that require shifting.

So be patient with yourself as you let go of the old toxic you and move into the new vibrant you!

THE TABLE HAS BEEN SET

I'd like to share with you the words I was given some years ago, just before opening the doors of my vegetarian restaurant called Vegitable. In the year before it opened, the world as I knew it had truly passed away: I went through a divorce, met and then lost the love of my life and his baby, and my mother—my best friend—died of cancer in my home. Then, the U.S. declared war in Afghanistan.

About a month before my restaurant was to open, I needed some retreat time for myself; so, I decided to take a trip overseas. The contractor I had hired to work on my restaurant was paid in full before I left, agreeing to have the entire place finished and the doors ready to open upon my return. When I arrived home, nothing had been done, and he was nowhere to be found. I was shocked, and in disbelief that anyone could do something like this to another human being. It was a bleak time, indeed, yet for me it ended up being the darkest hour before my dawn.

With tears streaming down my face, I dropped to my knees in prayer and heard these words:

Your mission is to help people get their physical bodies ready for the change that is now occurring on planet Earth. You are to set the table! Meditate upon these words and your doors will open!

Though the road that you travel may seem to bend and turn. Know my saints are there with you—these bends are so you'll learn.

The world as you've known it; it is passing away. In its destruction know I am there with you each and every day.

As your mission unfolds in the midst of war—look not to the left, nor to the right, but keep your eyes on my face and see what it is there for...for these wars and these rumors of wars, they're within each of us.

Fill your heart with love and watch! Ashes to ashes and dust to dust.

For the old is now passing with each breath that we take. The New Earth is emerging; this world has to shake!

Teaching divine love through the foods that you eat. Bringing people into your home and washing their feet.

For this bread, it is my body, take eat and remember me. This drink, it is my blood, drink it with love.

This table has been set for all those who see. Your house will be filled, the people, they are longing to be set free. Set free from the belief that they have been separated from Me.

—Christ, the light of the world!

In that moment, I was given the understanding that plant foods hold a power and purpose beyond scientific understanding. Through the power of photosynthesis, plant foods are infused with various colors of light. Therefore, when we eat plant foods, we are literally eating *The Body of Christ!*

Now this is true communion! Furthermore, I did successfully open the door to my restaurant, and we were a huge success!

In writing this book and sharing my story, I feel as though I am inviting you to not only sit at my table, but ultimately to sit at The Table of Christ, to commune around the idea of your body as a temple, and plant foods an offering—first as a reminder of your oneness with God, nature, the earth, and everyone around you, and then to serve you in remembering who and what you truly are!

My heartfelt prayer is that what I have given you within these pages is speaking to the answers you seek.

A CALL TO ACTION

As stated, food has both purpose and a power—to help you remember who and what you really are, and to prepare your body for the shift of the ages. So let the foods of light, air, water, and plants support you in creating a healthy, vibrant internal environment in alignment with the new world that is emerging.

From the new perspective of your body as an internal environment, these are among the most important ways to prepare yourself:

1. Monitor your first morning saliva pH regularly;
2. Educate yourself about the simple, ecological nature of life and how to thrive within the web of creation;
3. Stay attuned to the ever-changing modes of deception in agriculture, food, and medicine, and focus on how to make the evolutionary shift back to an ecotarian lifestyle. Join others in reversing this tide.
4. Stop eating the wrong kinds of S.O.S.—Salt, Oil, and Sugar;
5. Eat a plant-based diet only. Become "the light of the world!"
6. Move toward the alkaline end of the scale through the development of a new relationship with the sun, the air, and water.
7. Connect with your own internal physician and work daily with these four powerful "medicines" of air, fire, earth, and water, to banish any signs of disease and death.
8. Become an Internal Environmentalist by re-establishing ecological equilibrium within yourself and others.

Then, keep this mantra seated at the forefront of your mind:

The more I say YES! to life and living foods, the more life will say YES! to me.

THE POWER OF ONE

Perhaps you think it is all fine and good to restore your internal environment, but you should probably be out there picketing Monsanto or something, right? And then you sigh. If you have the desire to be an activist, that is a wonderful thing, but it isn't necessary in order for you to have great influence. Turning your attention inward can be equally as powerful as picketing, so can "demonstrating" with your wallet. If enough of us stop purchasing toxic foods, they eventually will be removed from our grocery shelves.

There is a paradox in that we think of our "self" as an individual unit, yet we are made up of numerous parts. You can think of the basic structure of our physical body as similar to the popular gift from the Soviet and other Eastern European countries—the nested Russian doll, a set of wooden dolls of decreasing size placed one inside the other.

Within the internal environment of the body at the most basic level we are atoms and molecules; from atoms and molecules are built the worlds of the cells; then larger systems such as skeletal, muscular, circulatory, organ and glandular, etc. are built from cellular structures; and finally those systems function together for the whole, integrated, enclosed landscape. However, within our entire body, there are trillions of microorganisms—even more than cells—that work synergistically so that we can function as a whole. However, most of our attention is focused on this magnificently enclosed environment as one functioning unit; we stand up and walk, talk, breathe, and live life as a relatively conscious individual—aware, yet unaware—of our inner workings.

As individuals, we are nested within our local communities, grouped in systems of gender, age, race, class, nation, culture, religion, etc., and then ultimately as members of the species of *homo sapiens,* or humans. As humans, we are just one of countless species living within the environment of planet Earth that is fully dependent on the continual stream of radiance from our great sun. You could say, perhaps, that we are all, ultimately, expressions of the sun.

Beyond this, there's our solar system's place within the cosmos, and the power of the creator that imbues it.

But what if size or perceived order doesn't really matter? What if every level of nesting—from the microscopic to the cosmic—is *equally* significant? What if the world of a short-lived cell is of equal power and significance to that of a long-lived planet, within the greater scheme of things? Moreso, what if these elements are inextricably linked meaning that one cannot survive without the other?

All of this is to say that the mind, the heart, and the actions of one person may be as important, and potentially as influential, as a galaxy. Are you beginning to comprehend the probability of how important (and magnificent) your internal ecosystems really are, and how much influence you really have?

If you feel like you don't have much confidence in your ability to impact the society or the healing of the earth through external action, then start by letting your influence be known in the internal world of your own body! And then see what happens.

THE INVISIBLE INFLUENCE OF YOUR DIET

There is a groundswell forming. We are at the cusp of change. We are moving into *ecotarian times*—eating and living a lifestyle that supports the sustainability of our bodies and planet. I feel so excited about the ecotarian evolutionary consciousness that is beginning to flower within us all. Just take a look at the book titles that are popping up on bookshelves now.

> *The Earth Diet, The Global Warming Diet, The Kind Diet, Diet for a New America: How Your Food Choices Affect Your Health, Happiness and the Future of Life on Earth, The Food Revolution: How Your Diet Can Help Save Your Life and Our World, The Good Food Revolution, Healthy Eating, Healthy World, Food Consciousness: A Food Relationship Revolution.*

Everywhere, people are making the connections between our diet, our relationship with food, and the life and health of the earth. This new trend is like the sliver of a new moon, but it will grow larger. Dietary devolution cannot continue; it has to change.

Because we are at a critical juncture on this earth, every decision we make has heightened consequences. Let's take a brief look at the four *fuel groups* that sustain us and how they are affected by our dietary choices.

The sun. It would seem like at least the sun is safe from human destruction. But there are a few who have ideas about using the sun as a disposal site for nuclear waste, so maybe it's not! At least for now, so far as we know, the source of the radiance of the sun remains untouched by human contamination.

However, all things work together. Polluted air and polluted waters can alter and block the pristine radiance of the sun. This is the case in both the environment of the earth and in our internal environment. To fully utilize the health-giving properties of the sun, living beings—both plants and animals—should receive it filtered through a clean atmosphere, and receive its life-giving charge through clean waters. Similarly, within the environment of the body, we are more capable of fully utilizing the radiance of the sun when the light that shines upon the waters of our body are free of toxic wastes.

So, do our dietary choices affect the air and the water? Yes, and mainly because of agricultural practices, as you will read about now.

The air. Rising levels of nitrogen-containing compounds, carbon dioxide and methane are driving the acidification of the atmosphere and, hence, global warming. The greatest producers of these gases are modern practices in livestock and agricultural production.

Here is just a glimpse at the problem. Ammonia, nitrogen nitrogen-containing compound, is the primary component of synthetic nitrogen fertilizers. Nitrous oxides are released in the burning of fossil fuels during the manufacturing of this fertilizer and other materials utilized in the production of the foods that we consume.

Alan Durning and John Ryan of the Northwest Environment Watch say the U.S. economy consumes nearly a pound of ammonia for each person every day, mostly as nitrogen fertilizer. They add that one-quarter of the nitrogen fertilizer used in the United States is applied to corn eaten by livestock. Furthermore, even though ammonia is applied as a fertilizer to the soil, because it is gaseous, much of it actually ends up releasing directly into the atmosphere.

The burning of fossil fuels for agricultural purposes, including the transportation of foods across the country, creates huge releases of nitrous compounds into the atmosphere, and enormous amounts of carbon dioxide, too. These are the acidifying compounds that are most responsible for acid rain and the acidification of rivers and oceans as fallout from the atmosphere. While carbonic acid fallout from carbon dioxide emissions is a serious concern, the global-warming potential of nitrous oxide is over 300 times greater. A parallel might be drawn to feeding the wrong fuels into the body: grain- and sugar-based foods create carbonic acid, while the digestion of meat creates nitrogenous acids.

Another potent greenhouse gas, methane, is produced in high amounts by livestock— yes, as flatulence! It might sound funny, but in fact, the levels of these toxic methane gasses in the atmosphere have tripled in the last century.

While atmospheric warming is a widespread phenomenon in our solar system right now, human dietary practices are adding their own pathological acid edge to the warming phenomenon on Earth, in more ways than you might imagine. For example, if a person's actions are creating an internal environment that is acidic, it is extremely likely that their actions toward their outer environment are the same, whether by critical, aggressive and even violent tendencies toward others, or unconscious choices that result in negativity within them, their family and the community.

This is why I so strongly endorse Mahatma Gandhi's words to *"be the change you wish to see in the world!"*

Consider doing your part to help the earth move through this transformative period of time. Consider making a commitment for just 90 days to no longer eat meat or dairy products! Significantly increase the amount of organic fruits and vegetables you eat. See for yourself how this makes you feel. Then take the next step and stop eating grains and beans for 90 days! See how this feels. Significantly increase the amount of fruit you eat.

Albert Einstein, the brilliant scientist who saw so deeply into the nature of things both great and small, saw the light already generations ago, when he said:

> *Nothing will benefit human health and increase chances for survival of life on Earth as much as the evolution to a vegetarian diet.*

While I agree, I'd like to take Albert Einstein's quote another step higher:

> **Nothing will benefit the sustainability of the human body and planet as much as the evolution into an ecotarian diet.**

The water. Modern practices in dairy and beef production facilities require tremendous amounts of water. According to soil and water specialists at the University of California Agricultural Extension, it takes about 5,200 gallons to produce 1 pound of beef.

In *The Food Revolution,* John Robbins makes this comparison: Let's say you take a 7 minute shower every single day, with a flow rate of 2 gallons per minute. At that rate, you would use 5,200 gallons of water to shower every day for *a year.*

You might think, well, the water used to produce meat doesn't disappear it just flows back into the Earth's hydrological system, right? Sure, but that's like saying it doesn't matter where your blood is in the body, as long as it's somewhere. Wrong!

Most of the water pumped from underground aquifers or diverted from rivers and lakes for livestock and dairy production is polluted in its use. Eventually, that polluted water ends up in streams, rivers, and finally the ocean, where it creates acidification and dead zones, and is no longer easily available for our use.

We are separating pure, fresh waters from the land at an increasing rate—much faster than they can be replaced. And even as the aquifers are gradually replenished by rainfall and seepage through the soils, in agricultural areas, they are replenished by nitrate-contaminated waters.

The earth. The location of livestock and poultry manures matters too. Animal manure is essential for the re-fertilization of the soil, but concentrated amounts of manure from forced animal containment systems end up contaminating soil and water. Vast expanses of land that were once renewed by the wastes of grazing ("free-range") animals are now saturated with poisonous chemicals instead, and topsoil's are being degraded and lost. Ryan and Durning figure that the production of every quarter-pound hamburger causes the loss of five times the burger's weight in topsoil.

It doesn't have to be this way. Our ancestors farmed very differently. Organic farming can be done in a way that sustains the health of soils, ecosystems, and people. And it can be economically sustainable. A research study undertaken by the Center for Biological Systems at Washington University in St. Louis concluded, "A five-year average shows that the organic farms yielded, in dollars per acre, exactly the same returns [as the chemical approach]."

But there's one more thing to consider. Our food choices not only affect the four elements and numerous non-human species of life, they affect other humans too! John Robbins, in *The Food Revolution,* provides these surprising and astonishing statistics.

- Number of underfed and malnourished people in the world: 1.2 billion.
- Number of overfed and malnourished people in the world: 1.2 billion.
- Experiences shared by both the hungry and the overweight: High levels of sickness and disability, shortened life expectancies, lower levels of productivity.
- Children in Bangladesh who are so underfed and underweight that their health is diminished: 56 percent.
- Adults in the United States who are so overfed and overweight that their health is diminished: 55 percent.

These statistics seem to point to the reality that we are *one* interdependent cosmos, affected simultaneously by the laws of science. Do your dietary choices affect humanity, animals and the earth? Are these choices significant? Indeed. Our food choices create the demand that generates the supply. In choosing an ecotarian diet for ourselves and our families, we are participating in the creation of a more sustainable agriculture and an ecologically sustainable world.

If you can't bear to go "cold turkey," you might consider at least starting by joining the Meatless Monday movement. Go one day a week without eating meat. If you can go one day, perhaps you can go two and then three ...

CHANGING OUR HABITS, ONE BITE AT A TIME

The challenge I had when first changing my diet was not the overwhelming temptation for a quick bite at a fast-food restaurant, but my mother's Sunday brunch. We had a large family, so tables lined with plates of food were set everywhere. My mother loved to cook and she created, by far, the best food I had ever eaten. But I loved myself more than I wanted to please her or my siblings, so I began to bring my own food. Needless to say, this was met with some resistance—at first.

While it took my mother time to adjust to my new way of eating, she saw the change in me and slowly began making changes herself. I had influenced her and the entire family, just by living the *EcoDiet* principles I had learned.

Instead of pot roast, ham, mashed potatoes, gravy, scrambled eggs, bacon, biscuits, meat-based casseroles, and lots of sugary desserts, she now served mounds of roasted vegetables, rosemary potatoes, scrumptious fruit and vegetable salads, and the best vegetarian casseroles I had ever eaten. Sunday brunches were no longer acidifying; they were alkalizing.

Change was in the air!

Not only did my entire family become healthier and happier, everyone started losing weight. They, too, were becoming the alkaline people they were designed to be!

The only question now is *are you ready*?

I am inclined to believe, since you've read this far, that you are...how exciting! You now hold the keys to life and health, or disease and death in your hand. Health is *your* choice. So why not choose it now? Make a choice today to join the *Ecotarian Revolution*, and to begin living the life you were designed to live as an ecotarian; and then choose it again and again, each and every day.

More and more people are joining hands with us to "be the change that we want to see in the world," and to experience our full potential as human beings on this magnificent planet. I hope with all my heart that you will join us on this incredible journey!

With love,

Toni Toney

AFTERWORD
by James Menzel Joseph

Toni Toney brings us shattering new possibilities for creative, exciting, health-filled tomorrows.

Imagine what your life and all life on our planet would be like if we were to live the principals and ideas set forth in, *EcoDiet*.

This book is a radical guide that goes to the root of our individual wellness, as well as to our collective human survival and that of all life in this ecosphere.

The broad based, well researched information within these pages is an inspiring guide for reconnecting to our innate oneness with all of life: as these insights unfold, they bring us a vision of what is possible in our lives.

We begin to see our interdependence, that this vast interdependent web of life is inseparable from our own lives. We see that life at its best is about experiencing wholeness—dissolving illusions of separation, or at least exploring that possibility in our moment to moment experiences.

Toni Toney has pulled back the curtain of misinformation and disinformation that is threatening our very existence as individuals and as a living world community. Through her extensive research into human physiology, she quickly lays many of our assumptions and beliefs to rest, the *things that everyone knows are true.* Then, she gives us a vision of *who we really are,* buried beneath the denial of our true physiology, the denial promoted by agribusiness, dietitians and the food processing industry, as well as other predatory interests that mould and shape our "reality." This denial of who we really are has us suffering from diseases of epidemic proportion—heart disease, diabetes and cancer, to name only the most obvious. Our bodies, minds and spirits are crying out for our awakening from this deadly trance, this dance of planetary death impatiently awaiting our rebirth.

We are offered, within these pages, the opportunity to live in a body that is fully alive and awake...urging us to become that person who is up to the challenge of creating new realities—realities that are sweeping away our commonly held assumptions, and *the dysfunctional and dangerous beliefs that now threaten our very survival, both personally and globally.* Are we up to the possibility of being healers, for ourselves, our loved ones, and for our planet? Toni Toney has shown us the way, in this beautiful tribute to what is possible through a relentless search for a sustaining truth. Through her perseverance she has brought us new possibilities for creative, exciting and health filled tomorrows.

In a very real sense, this book carries the seed of a profound revolution—a revolution without guns and banners; a revolution that turns one lawn at a time into a garden, one corn field into an orchard, and one suffering person, turned healthy. You and I are its army—an army of wellness, a potentially growing army with people who have discovered, recovered our life sustaining essence. *It is our celebratory passion born of this newfound awareness that can resuscitate our deeply troubled ecosphere, person by inspired person.*

Toni Toney shatters many of our assumptions about who we really are physiologically: what we thought was essential to our well-being is brought into question or, often, simply swept away. *EcoDiet* illuminates us as well to our abuse of land and animals, and how starvation among our suffering fellow humans due to our carnivore appetites can be greatly reduced by our personal choices. This helps us see that the ecological nightmare of deforestation can also be dissolved to be replaced by lush and verdant gardens—gardens that would bring oxygen to the now dead and denuded land; land regenerated by fruit and nut trees. The aroma of living plants, blossoms and spices would fill the air instead of that of the morbid stench of feedlots.

We can choose to stop eating high on the food chain; stop inflicting pain and suffering on other sentient beings; stop the clearing of rain forests to raise cattle; stop the ten pounds of grain needed for every pound of meat produced; and stop the poisoning of our air, waters and streams. By eating living foods we are more likely to become inspired, vibrant and alive: we see that life is much more than the sum of its parts... No, it's the whole, the *Holy*...

The only way life can be fully understood and fully appreciated is by getting back in touch with our essence.

EcoDiet *brings us back in touch with a sense of wholeness and away from the sense of alienation so pervasive in our culture today.*

Thank you Toni Toney for sharing your iconoclastic and penetrating vision. May we all join together in conscious, loving action toward creating the world that we truly wish to see.

J. Menzel-Joseph, Artist, Writer, Teacher and
Author of *Art & Survival in the Twenty-first Century*
and the soon to be published *The Transcending Heart...*
Imaginings from beyond the Mind

REFERENCE NOTES

Chapter 1: How I Almost Died

Al Gore, An Inconvenient Truth: The Crisis of Global Warming, rev ed (New York: Viking, 2007); and <www.climatecrisis.net>, the official site for the film An Inconvenient Truth, featuring Al Gore (Paramount, 100 min, 2006). See the book and film for powerful insights into the nature of global warming.

James Lovelock, The Revenge of Gaia: Earth's Climate Crisis & the Fate of Humanity (New York: Basic Books, 2006).

HIPPOCRATES: THE FATHER OF MEDICINE

For the medical philosophy of Hippocrates (460–377 BCE), see Ann Wigmore, The Hippocrates Diet and Health Program: A Natural Diet and Health Program for Weight Control, Disease Prevention, and Life Extension (New York: Avery Trade, 1983).

THE INTERNAL TERRAIN THEORY

Nancy Appleton, The Curse of Louis Pasteur: Why Medicine Is Not Healing a Diseased World (Santa Monica: Choice Publishing, 1999). A portrait of the lives of Béchamp and Pasteur and their contrasting theories.

Christopher Bird, "To Be or Not to Be? 150 Years of Hidden Knowledge," Nexus Magazine, April 1992. An introduction to the internal terrain theory and the amazing habits of microzymas.

"Biological Terrain vs. the Germ Theory," The Health Advantage, <http://thehealthadvantage.com/biologicalterrain.html>.

Antoine Béchamp, The Third Element of the Blood, trans Montague R Leverson (1911; Collingwood, Vic: Zigguart, 1994).

Bernard Jensen and Mark Anderson, Empty Harvest (1990; repr, New York: Avery, 1995).

Christopher Bird, The Life and Trials of Gaston Naessens: The Galileo of the Microscope (St. Lambert, Quebec: Les Presses de l'Université de la Personne, 1990), p 31.

THE GERM: THE CAUSE, THE CURE

Deanna M Minich, PhD, FACN, CNS, Jeffrey S Bland, PhD, FACN, "Acid-Alkaline Balance: Role in Chronic Disease and Detoxification," Alternative Therapies 13, no 4 (2007).

Albert Einstein, letter of 1950, as quoted in The New York Times (March 29, 1972) and The New York Post (Nov 28, 1972).

Chapter 2: Our Body Is a Living Ecosystem

PRIMARY CONSUMER ORGANISMS: FRUGIVORES

Katherine Milton, "Diet and Primate Evolution," Scientific American, Aug 1993: 86–93, <http://nature.berkeley.edu/miltonlab/pdfs/diet_primate_evolution.pdf>.

Karen B Strier, Primate Behavioral Ecology (Boston: Pearson Allyn and Bacon, 2007).

Christopher Ryan and Cacilda Jethá, Sex at Dawn: How We Mate, Why We Stray, and What It Means for Modern Relationships, (New York: Harper, 2010).

EAT RIGHT FOR YOUR ANATOMICAL TYPE

Frances Moore Lappé, Diet for a Small Planet (1971; New York: Ballantine, 1991), p. 12.

Cardiologist William C Roberts, editor in chief of The American Journal of Cardiology and medical director of the Baylor Heart and Vascular Institute at Baylor University Medical Center in Dallas, is cited in Sally Deneen, "Body of Evidence: Were Humans Meant to Eat Meat?" E/The Environmental Magazine 13, no 1 (Jan/Febr 2002), <www.emagazine.com>.

Robert Morse, ND, The Detox Miracle Sourcebook (Prescott, AZ: Hohm Press, 2004), pp 8–11. Dr. Morse operates a natural health clinic in Florida, specializing in brain and nerve regeneration. See his website at <http://www.drmorsesherbalhealth club.com/>.

Victoria Boutenko, Green for Life (Ashland, OR: Raw Family Pub, 2005), p. 11.

Chapter 3: Unnatural Feeding Causes Ecological Breakdowns

HOW BODIES OF WATER THRIVE OR DIE

Peter Montague, "Pollution of World's Largest Lakes Shows Importance of Banning Toxics," Environmental Research Foundation publication 146 (1989), <www.rachel.org>.

Doug Jeanneret, "Lake Erie Water Quality: Past, Present and Future," Fact Sheet 046 (Columbus, OH: Ohio Sea Grant College Program, 1989), <http://www.sg.ohio-state.edu/publications/water/fs-046.html>.

Spencer Hunt, "Algae, Invaders Threaten Lake Erie," The Columbus Dispatch, Nov 25, 2012, <http://www.dispatch.com/content/stories/local/2012/11/25/algae-invaders-threaten-lake-erie.html>.

HOW WE THRIVE OR DIE

Martha M Grout, MD, MD(H), "Inflammation," Arizona Center for Advanced Medicine, 2007, <http://www.arizonaadvancedmedicine.com/articles/inflammation.html>.

CANDIDA: THE SILENT KILLER

Josep Guarro, Josepa Gené, and Alberto M Stchigel, "Developments in Fungal Taxonomy," Clin Microbiol Rev 12, no 3 (July 1999): 454–500.

Candida Yeast Infection Self Exams, National Candida Center, <http://www.national candidacenter.com/candida-self-exams/>.

DIABETES: THE CAUSE, THE CURE

Douglas N Graham, DC, The 80/10/10 Diet (Key Largo, FL: FoodnSport Press, 2006), p. 38.

Neal D Barnard, MD, Neal Barnard's Program for Reversing Diabetes (New York: Rodale, 2007).

Patrick Schrauwen, "Highfat Diet, Muscular Lipotoxicity and Insulin Resistance," Proceedings of the Nutrition Society 66 (2007), 33–41, doi: 10.1017/S0029665107005277.

John McDougall, MD, interview by Dennis Hughes, <http://www.shareguide.com/McDougall.html>.

CANCER: THE CAUSE, THE CURE

Tullio Simoncini, MD, Cancer Is a Fungus (Rome, Italy: Edizioni Lampis, 2007), <www.cancerisafungus.com>.

Otto Warburg, "The Prime Cause and Prevention of Cancer," (Lecture delivered to Nobel Laureates at Lindau, by Lake Constance, Germany, on June 30, 1966), trans and ed by Dean Burk, National Cancer Institute, p 6. Otto Warburg was the director of the Max Planck Institute for Cell Physiology, Berlin, Germany. He was the recipient of two Nobel Prizes and many other awards and honors for his work in the chemistry and physics of life. Retrieved from <www.ozonetherapy.co.uk>.

Stephen Levine, PhD, and Parris M Kidd, PhD, "Beyond Antioxidant Adaptation: A Free Radical-Hypoxia-Clonal Thesis of Cancer Causation," Journal of Orthomolecular Psychiatry 14, no 3 (1985): 189–213.

Hiromi Shinya, MD, The Microbe Factor (San Francisco: Council Oak Books, LLC, 2010), p 52.

Prof Dr Gunther Enderlein, Blood Examination in Darkfield, monographs summarized and trans by Dr med Maria-M Bleker (Germany: Semmelweis Verlag, 1993), p 11.

"Oxygen Therapies: Interview with Ed McCabe," by Stuart Ledbetter, Nexus Magazine, Aug–Sept, 1992. Adapted from an interview of Ed McCabe on NBC affiliate WPTZ Television, Plattsburgh, NY, <http://www.whale.to/v/mccabe1.html>.

Chapter 4: The Internal Acid Rain Theory

HOW ACID RAIN DESTROYS OUR PLANET

The image of the acid-rain cycle is archived at <http://www.oocities.org/energyconsumption/acidrain.html>.

HOW ACID RAIN DESTROYS AQUATIC ECOSYSTEMS

Paul Withers, "New Culprit Identified in Chronic Acid Rain Problem," CBC News (Nova Scotia), Nov 23, 2012, <http://www.cbc.ca/news/canada/nova-scotia/story/2012/11/22/ns-acid-rain.html>.

Marissa Weiss, "Is Acid Rain a Thing of the Past?" June 28, 2012, <http://news.sciencemag.org/sciencenow/2012/06/is-acid-rain-a-thing-of-the-past.html>.

Tristan Jones, "Energy, Agriculture, and the Environment: Dead Zones and the Oil Spill in the Gulf of Mexico," June 22, 2010, <http://blogs.ei.columbia.edu/2010/06/22/energy-agriculture-and-the-environment-dead-zones-and-the-oil-spill-in-the-gulf-of-mexico/>.

VALIDATION OF THE INTERNAL ACID RAIN THEORY

Garth L Nicolson, PhD, "Chronic Bacterial and Viral Infections in Neurodegenerative and Neurobehavioral Diseases," Medscape, posted June 23, 2008, <http://www.medscape.com/viewarticle/574944>.

Lorne Label, MD, personal communication, 1998. Dr. Label is associate clinical professor of neurology at the David Geffen School of Medicine at UCLA, adjunct faculty at Loyola Marymount University, medical director of both the Southern California Attention Deficit Disorder Clinic and the Brain Longevity Center, and is in private practice with California Neurological Specialists, where he practices adult and pediatric neurology and medical acupuncture.

Pogo is the title and central character of a comic strip created by Walt Kelly (1913–1973).

Chapter 5: How to Conduct an Internal Acid Rain Study

MT Morter, Jr, Correlative Urinalysis: The Body Knows Best (Rogers, AR: B.E.S.T. Research Inc, 1987). I have often relied on the superlative wisdom and clarity of Dr. MT Morter, Jr, with regards to pH and the acid/alkaline balance. Dr. Morter is a great researcher, teacher, and mentor, whose understanding of the body and the ramifications of the acid/alkaline balance never ceases to amaze me. See Correlative Urinalysis, especially pp 31–36, for a more in-depth discussion of buffering systems and the interpretation of test results. For a general guide to acid and alkaline ash–forming foods, see Dr. Morter's Your Health, Your Choice: Your Complete Personal Guide to Wellness, Nutrition and Disease Prevention (Hollywood, FL: Fell Publishers, 1990).

Robert R Barefoot and Carl J Reich, MD, The Calcium Factor: the Scientific Secret of Health and Youth (Wickenburg, AZ: Pan American International Nutrition Ltd, 2006).

Hippocrates, Epidemics, <http://ancienthistory.about.com/od/greekmedicine/f/HippocraticOath.htm>.

Chapter 6: It's Time to Stop the Dietary Devolution Movement

DIETARY DEVOLUTION #1
FROM FRUGIVORE TO OMNIVORE
Boyce Rensberger, "Research Yields Surprises about Early Human Diets: Teeth Show Fruit Was the Staple," New York Times, May 15, 1979.

Hilton Hotema, Man's Higher Consciousness (Kessinger Publishing, 1962).

Anthony Sebastian, "Estimation of the Net Acid Load of the Diet of Ancestral Preagricultural Homo Sapiens and their Hominid Ancestors," American Journal of Clinical Nutrition 76, no 6 (Dec 2002): 1308–16.

WE ARE NOT DESIGNED TO EAT GRAINS

Arnold Ehret, Mucusless Diet Healing System (1922; repr., Dobbs Ferry, NY: Ehret Literature Publishing Co, 1994).

Rhonda Nelson, PhD, Diagnos-Techs, Inc. Lab, Gluten Intolerance Seminar, 2012, as reported by JoAnn Newton on her webpage <http://www.joannnewton.com/blog/2012/06/28/Gluten-Intolerance.aspx>.

Kaayla Daniel, PhD, CCN, "Plants Bite Back," Wise Traditions in Food, Farming and the Healing Arts, the quarterly magazine of the Weston A Price Foundation, Spring 2010, <http://www.westonaprice.org/Plants-Bite-Back.html>.

R Paul St Amand and Claudia Marek, What Your Doctor may Not Tell You about Fibromyalgia: The Revolutionary Treatment that Can Reverse the Disease (New York: Warner Books, 1999).

A Bengtsson, KG Henriksson, and J Larsson, "Reduced High-Energy Phosphate Levels in the Painful Muscles of Patients with Primary Fibromyalgia," Arthritis Rheum 29 (1986): 817–21.

Hertha Hafer, The Hidden Drug: Dietary Phosphate, trans Jane Donlin (Armadale: PHOSADD Australia, 2001).

Lendon H Smith, MD, "ADHD and ADD: The Hyperactive Child," <http://www.phosadd.com/support%20evidence/lsmith.htm>.

BUT WHERE DO I GET MY PROTEIN?

Deborah E Sellmeyer, Katie L Stone, Anthony Sebastian, Steven R Cummings, and the Study of Osteoporotic Fractures Research Group, UNC-SF, "A High Ratio of Dietary Animal to Vegetable Protein Increases the Rate of Bone Loss and the Risk of Fracture in Postmenopausal Women," American Journal of Clinical Nutrition 73, no 1 (Jan 2001): 118–22.

T Colin Campbell, PhD, with Thomas M Campbell II, The China Study: Startling Implications for Diet, Weight Loss and Long-term Health (Dallas, TX: BenBella Books, 2005), introduction and pp 58-59.

Jane E. Brody, "Huge Study of Diet Indicts Fat and Meat," New York Times, May 8, 1990.

Rob Stein, "Daily Red Meat Raises Chances of Dying Early," Washington Post, March 24, 2009.

Paul Jaminet, "Pork: Did Leviticus 11:7 Have It Right?" Parts 1-3, February 8–22, 2012, <http://perfecthealthdiet.com>.

WANT TO SAVE OUR PLANET?
STOP EATING MEAT!

The Livestock, Environment, and Development Initiative, Livestock's Long Shadow: Environmental Issues and Options (Food and Agriculture Organization of the United Nations [FAO], 2006), <ftp://ftp.fao.org/docrep/fao/010/a0701e/a0701e.pdf>.

DIETARY DEVOLUTION #2: FROM OMNIVORE TO CHEMIVORE
HOW CHEMICALS ENTER THE FOOD CHAIN

Marla Cone, "Ancestral Diet Gone Toxic," Los Angeles Times, January 13, 2004, A-1, <http://articles.latimes.com/2004/jan/13/local/me-inuit13>.

WANT TO LOSE WEIGHT?
STOP EATING TOXIC MEAT

Paula Baillie-Hamilton, MD, PhD, The Body Restoration Plan: Eliminate Chemical Calories and Repair Your Body's Natural Slimming System (New York: Penguin, 2002). This is a little-known but truly valuable resource.

WANT TO AVOID CANCER?
CUT OUT THE COLD CUTS

Amanda J Cross , Michael F Leitzmann, Mitchell H Gail, Albert R Hollenbeck, Arthur Schatzkin, Rashmi Sinha, "A Prospective Study of Red and Processed Meat Intake in Relation to Cancer Risk," PLoS Med 4, no 12 (2007): e325. doi: 10.1371/journal. pmed.0040325.

CS Bruning-Fann, JB Kaneene, "The Effects of Nitrate, Nitrite, and N-nitroso Compounds on Human Health: A Review," Vet Human Toxicology 35 (1993): 521–38.

STOP EATING FROM TOXIC OCEANS
Alicia Chang, "Radioactive Bluefin Tuna: Japan Nuclear Plant Contaminated Fish Found off California Coast," Huffington Post, May 28, 2012.

Michael Collins, "Japanese Seaweed Radiation Doubles," April 20, 2012, <Enviro Reporter.com>.

Environmental Working Group, "Brain Food: Government Seafood Consumption Advice Could Expose 1 in 4 Newborns to Elevated Mercury Levels," April 13, 2001, <http://www.ewg.org/book/export/html/8143>.

Ronald A Hites, Jeffery A Foran, David O Carpenter, M Coreen Hamilton, Barbara A Knuth, Steven J Schwager, "Global Assessment of Organic Contaminants in Farmed Salmon," Science 303, no 5655 (2004): 226–29, doi: 10.1126/science.1091447.

Kristen Schmitt, "Wild No More: Farm-Raised Fish labeled as 'Wild Caught'," UrbanTimes, April 23, 2012, <http://www.theurbn.com/2012/04/wild-no-more-farm-raised-fish-labeled-as-wild-caught/>.

STOP CONSUMING DAIRY PRODUCTS
See the many articles on the dangers of milk at <www.notmilk.com>.
Linda Joyce Forristal, CTA, MTA, "Ultra-Pasteurized Milk," May 23, 2004, <www.motherlindas.com>.

Keith B Woodford, Devil in the Milk: Illness, Health and Politics of A1 and A2 Milk (White River Junction, VT: Chelsea Green Pub, 2009).

William Campbell Douglass II, MD, The Raw Truth about Milk, rev and expanded ed (Douglass Family Pub: 2007).

STOP EATING FOOD FROM TOXIC FIELDS

Joe Cummins, "Bt Toxins in Genetically Modified Crops: Regulation by Deceit," Institute of Science in Society, March 23, 2004, <http://www.i-sis.org.uk/BTTIGMC.php>.

Richard Pressinger, MEd, and Wayne Sinclair, MD, "Researching Effects of Chemicals and Pesticides upon Health," <http://www.chem-tox.com/>.

Paula Baillie-Hamilton, MD, The Body Restoration Plan (New York: Penguin, 2002).

THE GROWING PROBLEM OF MYCOTOXINS

Charles M Benbrook, Chief Scientist, The Organic Center, "Breaking the Mold: Impacts of Organic and Conventional Farming Systems on Mycotoxins in Food and Livestock Feed," Sept2006, <www.organic-center.org/reportfiles/MycotoxinReport.pdf>.

Don Huber, Transcript of interview by Dr. Joseph Mercola, Jan 2012, <http://mercola.fileburst.com/PDF/ExpertInterviewTranscripts/InterviewDonHuber-Part2.pdf>.

Dave Asprey, "The Molding of the World Part 1: How We Made Mycotoxins into the Health Disaster They Are Today," March 22, 2012, <http://www.bulletproofexec.com/mycotoxins-in-america/>.

WANT PRODUCE WITH LOTS OF NUTRIENTS?
EAT ORGANIC

For the Biodynamic Farming and Gardening Association, see <www.biodynamics.com>.

Catharine Paddock, "Organic Food Is More Nutritious Say EU Researchers," Medical News Today, Oct 29, 2007, <http://www.medicalnewstoday.com/articles/86972.php>.

Steve Diver, "Nutritional Quality of Organically Grown Food," ATTRA, Revised 2002, <http://www.soilandhealth.org/06clipfile/nutritional%20quality%20of%20organically-grown%20food.html>.

STOP EATING IRRADIATED FOODS

Organic Consumers Association, "What's Wrong with Food Irradiation," Febr 2001, <http://www.organicconsumers.org/Irrad/irradfact.cfm>.

Organic Consumers Association, "Status Update on Food Irradiation," July 5, 2002, <http://www.organicconsumers.org/Irrad/status.cfm>.

STOP THE GMO DEVOLUTION MADNESS

"What Are the Dangers?" Mothers for Natural Law, <http://www.safe-food.org/-issue/dangers.html>.

"Arpad Pusztain and the Risks of Genetic Engineering," The Organic and Non-GMO Report, ed Ken Roseboro, 2009.

Joël Spiroux de Vendômois, Francois Roullier, Dominique Cellier, Gilles-Eric Séralini, "A Comparison of the Effects of Three GM Corn Varieties on Mammalian Health," Int J Biological Sciences 5, no 7 (2009): 706–26, doi: 10.7150/ijbs.5.706.

Rady Ananda, "Three Approved GMOs Linked to Organ Damage," Jan 3, 2012, <http://prn.fm/2012/01/03/foodfreedom-com-three-approved-gmos-linked-to-organ-damage/#axzz1wZmHPTF4>.

UNRAVELING THE GENETIC STRAND

Dag Falck, "Does the Current Organic Practice Standard Adequately Address GMO Contamination?" The Organic and Non-GMO Report, Jan 2008, <http://www.non-gmoreport.com/articles/jan08/organic_practice_standard_and_gmo_contamination.php>.

WANT TO AVOID GMOS?
EAT ORGANIC!

Barry Flamm, Chair of the National Organic Standards Board, "Open Letter from National Organic Standards Board to USDA on GMO Contamination of Organic Crops," March 28, 2012, <http://www.organicconsumers.org/articles/article_25217.cfm>.

DIETARY DEVOLUTION #3:FROM CHEMIVORE TO JUNKIVORE

Mary Forgione, "What Does 'Natural' Food Mean," Los Angeles Times, Nov 5, 2010, <http://articles.latimes.com/2010/nov/05/news/la-heb-natural-claims-food-20101105>.

Eric Schlosser, "Why McDonald's Fries Taste so Good," Jan 17, 2001, excerpt from Fast Food Nation (Houghton-Mifflin, 2001), <http://rense.com/general7/whyy.htm>.

STOP EATING EMPTY CALORIES

Mark Hyman, MD, "How Malnutrition Causes Obesity," Huffington Post, March 8, 2012, <http://www.huffingtonpost.com/dr-mark-hyman/malnutrition-obesity_b_1324760.html> and "Skinny Fat People: Why Being Skinny Doesn't Protect Us Against Diabetes and Death," May 22, 2012, <http://drhyman.com/blog/2012/05/22/skinny-fat-people-why-being-skinny-doesnt-protect-us-against-diabetes-and-death/>.

EATING MSG?
IF IT'S IN A BOX, YOU PROBABLY ARE!

K He, L Zhao, ML Daviglus, AR Dyer, L Van Horn, D Garside, L Zhu, D Guo, Y Wu, B Zhou, J Stamler; INTERMAP Cooperative Research Group, "Association of Monosodium Glutamate Intake with Overweight in Chinese Adults: the INTERMAP Study," Obesity (Silver Spring) 16, no 8 (2008): 1875–80.

ADDICTED TO FAKE SUGAR?
DITCH THE DIET DRINKS!

Janet Starr Hull, Creator of the Aspartame Detox Program, "Dangers of Aspartame Poisoning," 2002, <www.sweetpoison.com/aspartame-information.html>.

Theresa Dale, ND, "Aspartame: More Unsavory Side Effects," Spartan of Truth: Archive for Lendon Smith, MD, Dec 4, 2011, <http://spartanoftruth.wordpress.com/tag/lendon-smith-m-d/>.

Sandra Cabot, MD, "Aspartame Makes You Fatter!" Position Statement, July 22, 2006, <http://www.liverdoctor.com>.

FAKE FAT MAKES YOU FATTER!

Myra Karstadt and Stephen Schmidt, "Olestra: Procter's Big Gamble," CSPI Nutrition Action Health Letter, March 1996, <http://www.cspinet.org/olestra/pbg.html>.

Susan E Swithers, Sean B Ogden, Terry L Davidson, "Fat Substitutes Promote Weight Gain in Rats consuming high-fat diets," Behavioral Neuroscience 125, no 4 (Aug 2011): 512–18, doi: 10.1037/a0024404.

THE HIDDEN TRUTH ABOUT GMOS
WHAT MANUFACTURERS AREN'T TELLING YOU!

Relaena, "Is Organic Always GMO Free?" GMO Awareness, May 5, 2011, <http://gmo-awareness.com/2011/05/05/is-organic-always-gmo-free/>.

Michael Pollan, interview by Amy Goodman, Democracy Now, Oct 24, 2012. For a transcript see <http://www.democracynow.org/2012/10/24/michael_pollan_californias_prop_37_fight>.

THE LAKE ERIE SYNDROME

Hertha Hafer, Diet Connection, <http://www.phosadd.com/mainpage/main33.htm>.

Paula Baille-Hamilton, MD, The Body Restoration Plan, p 32.

CAN YOU AFFORD TO BE A JUNKAVORE?

Economic Research Service, Table 13: US Per Capita Food Expenditures, <http://www.ers.usda.gov/data-products/food-expenditures.aspx>.

David U Himmelstein, MD, Deborah Thorne, PhD, Elizabeth Warren, JD, Steffie Woolhandler, ND, MPH, "Medical Bankruptcy in the United States, 2007: Results of a National Study," American Journal of Medicine 20, no 10 (2009), doi: 10.1016/j.amjmed.2009.04.012.

DIETARY DEVOLUTION #4: FROM JUNKIVORE TO DRUGIVORE

Melinda Wenner, "Humans Carry More Bacterial Cells than Human Ones," Scientific American, Nov 30, 2007, <http://www.scientificamerican.com/article.cfm?id=strange-but-true-humans-carry-more-bacterial-cells-than-human-ones>.

HL Queen, Chronic Mercury Toxicity: New Hope Against an Endemic Disease (Colorado Springs, CO: Queen and Company Health Communications, 1988).

Bernard Jensen, DC, ND, PhD, Iridology: Science and Practice in the Healing Arts, Vol II (Escondido, CA: Bernard Jensen, 1982), p 436–37.

THE DEVOLUTION OF DISEASE

George J Armelagos, Kathleen C Barnes, and James Lin, "Disease in Human Evolution: The Re-Emergence of Infections Disease in the Third Epidemiological Transition," National Museum of Natural History Bulletin for Teachers 18, no 3 (Fall 1996).

Charles Dickens (1812–1870), A Tale of Two Cities.

Chapter 7: Has Your Body Been Sending You an S-O-S Signal?

THE WRONG TYPE OF SALT

Elizabeth Walling, "Unrefined Sea Salt vs. Table Salt," Aug 23, 2011, <http://www.celticseasaltblog.com/unrefined-sea-salt-vs-table-salt-by-elizabeth-walling/>.

"Iodized Salt," Salt Institute, <http://www.saltinstitute.org/Issues-in-focus/Food-salt-health/Iodized-salt-other-additives>.

THE RIGHT TYPE OF SALT

Selina, "The Missing Ingredients in the Salt Debate," Febr 1, 2011, <http://www.celticseasaltblog.com/the-missing-ingredients-in-the-salt-debate/>.

Barbara Hendel and Peter Ferreira, Water and Salt: The Essence of Life: The Healing Power of Nature (Natural Resources, 2003).

THE WRONG TYPE OF OIL

Ray Peat, "Unsaturated Vegetable Oils: Toxic," 2006, <http://raypeat.com/articles/articles/unsaturated-oils.shtml>. I drew heavily on this article, in which a great deal of information is brought together and summarized.

Paavo O Airola, Are You Confused? (Phoenix, AZ: Health Plus, 1971), p 96.

T Colin Campbell, PhD, with Thomas M Campbell II, The China Study, pp 69-90.

Caldwell B Esselstyn, Prevent and Reverse Heart Disease: The Revolutionary, Scientifically Proven Nutrition-Based Cure (New York: Avery, 2007).

Victoria Boutenko, "Green for Life Second Edition," Raw Family, <http://www.rawfamily.com/newsletters/green-for-life-2nd-edition>.

"Harvard Review of Evidence Verifies That Eating Trans Fats Increases Risk of Heart Disease," Harvard School of Public Health press release, June 23, 1999, <www.hsph.harvard.edu/news/press-releases/archives/1999-releasespress06231999.html>.

Fiona Haynes, "Do All Foods Listing Hydrogenated Oils Contain Trans Fats?" <http://lowfatcooking.about.com/od/faqs/f/hydrogenated.htm>.

Paul Jaminet, "Pork: Did Leviticus 11:7 Have It Right?".

THE RIGHT TYPE OF OIL
Stephan Guyenet, PhD, "Does Dietary Saturated Fat Increase Blood Cholesterol? An Informal Review of Observational Studies," Whole Health Source, Jan 13, 2011, <http://wholehealthsource.blogspot.com/2011/01/does-dietary-saturated-fat-increase.html>.

Ray Peat, "Coconut Oil," 2006, and "Unsaturated Fatty Acids: Nutritionally Essential, or Toxic?" 2007, <http://raypeat.com/articles/>.

Monica Eng, "Has Your Food Gone Rancid? Consumers May Have Kitchen Full of Dangerous Products and Not Know It," Chicago Tribune, March 7, 2012, <http://articles.chicagotribune.com/2012-03-07/features/sc-food-0302-rancidity-20120307_1_trans-fats-polyunsaturated-oils-food-chain>.

THE WRONG TYPE OF SUGAR
Robert H Lustig, Fat Chance: Beat the Odds Against Sugar, Processed Food, Obesity, and Disease (Penguin Group, 2013).

Mehmet Oz, expert answer to "How Much Sugar Does the Average Person Consume Every Year?" <http://www.sharecare.com/question/sugar-consume-every-year>.

Bill Sanda, "Double Dangers of High Fructose Corn Syrup," Wise Traditions in Food, Farming and the Healing Arts, Weston Price Foundation, Winter 2003.

Renee Dufault, Blaise LeBlanc, Roseanne Schnoll, Charles Cornett, Laura Schweitzer, David Wallinga, Jane Hightower, Lyn Patrick, and Walter J Lukiw, "Mercury from Chlor-Alkali Plants: Measured Concentrations in Food Product Sugar," Environmental Health 8, no 2 (2009), doi: 10.1186/1476-069X-8-2.

THE RIGHT TYPE OF SUGAR

Gabriel Cousins, MD, MD(H), "My 22 Most Recommended Food Energies," <http://www.cultureoflifestore.com/p3/Gabriel+Recommends/pages.html>.

Bryan Marcel, "Truvia and PureVia Are not Stevia," April 24, 2010, <http://www.bryanmarcel.com/truvia-and-purevia-are-not-stevia>.

Chapter 8: Stop Acidifying and Start Alkalizing

STRONGLY ACIDIFYING FOODS AND DRINKS

As in chapter 5, I've drawn on the wisdom of MT Morter, Jr, for my understanding of the effects of acidifying foods in the body.

Dave Asprey, "Why Bad Coffee Makes You Weak," Dec 20, 2011, <http://www.bulletproofexec.com/why-bad-coffee-makes-you-weak/>.

SOFT DRINKS

Mark Hyman, "Skinny Fat People."

Brett Israel, "Brominated Battle: Soda Chemical Has Cloudy Health History," Scientific American, Dec 12, 2011, <http://www.scientificamerican.com/article.cfm?id=soda-chemical-cloudy-health-history>.

Linda Larsen, "CSPI Finds 4-MI Levels in Coca-Cola Vary Worldwide," Food Poisoning Bulletin, June 27, 2012, <http://foodpoisoningbulletin.com/2012/cspi-finds-4-mi-levels-in-coca-cola-vary-worldwide/>.

Mike Adams, "Suffering from Soft Drinks," <http://www.bibliotecapleyades.net/ciencia/ciencia_industryweapons55.htm>, and The Five Soft Drink Monsters: How to Finally Kick the Soft Drink Habit for Good (Truth Pub, 2005).

SPORTS AND ENERGY DRINKS

Rob Faigin, "Rob Declares War on Gatorade," Rob Report #4, Febr 2, 2005, <http://www.extique.com/robreport-4.htm>.

John P Higgins, Troy D Tuttle, Christopher L Higgins, "Energy Beverages: Content and Safety," Mayo Clinic Proceedings 81, no 11 (Nov 2010): 1033–41.

Academy of General Dentistry and Stan Diel, "Energy Drinks are 10 Times Worse for Teeth than Colas," Dental Health Magazine, May 2, 2008, <http://worldental.org/nutrition/energy-drinks-bad-teeth/241/>.

Michael F Jacobson, executive director of CSPI, "Sunny Delight Is Designed to Deceive," April 24, 2002, <http://www.cspinet.org/new/sunny_042402.html>.

PLASTIC WATER

Executive Summary of Eric D Olson, Bottled Water: Pure Drink or Pure Hype? April 1999, <http://www.nrdc.org/water/drinking/bw/exesum.asp>.

F Grün and B Blumberg, "Endocrine Disrupters as Obesogens," Mol Cell Endocrinol 304, no 1–2 (May 2009): 19–29, doi: 10.1016/j.mce.2009.02.018.

MILDLY ACIDIFYING FOODS AND DRINKS

J Vinson, X Su, L Zubik, P Bose, "Phenol Antioxidant Quantity and Quality in Foods: Fruits," J Agric Food Chem 49, no 11 (Nov 2001): 5315–32.

"Studies Showing Adverse Effects of Dietary Soy, 1939–2008," Weston A Price Foundation, <http://www.westonaprice.org/soy-alert/studies-showing-adverse-effects-of-soy>.

Ellen Coleman, MA, MPH, RD, CSSD, "Dietary Fiber and Cardiovascular Disease," Nuturition Dimension, Continuing Education Module, 2011 Edition, <http://www.nutrition411.com/ce_pdf/DietaryFiberandCardiovascularDisease.pdf>.

Paul Pitchford, Healing with Whole Foods: Asian Traditions and Modern Nutriton (Berkeley, CA: North Atlantic Books, 2002), p 530.

The idea of berries as inoculators came from a conversation with Don Tolman, author of Farmacist Desk Reference (Park City, UT: Ynot Eduk8, 2007).

Guillaume Ruel, Msc, Sonia Pomerleau, RD, Msc, Patrick Couture, MD, PhD, Simone Lemieux, PhD, Benoît Lamarche, PhD, FAHA and Charles Couillard, PhD, "Plasma Matrix Metalloproteinase (MMP)-9 Levels Are Reduced Following Low-Calorie Cranberry Juice Supplementation in Men," J Am Coll Nutr 28, no 6 (Dec 2009): 694–701, <http://www.jacn.org/content/28/6/694>.

ACIDIFYING THOUGHTS AND EMOTIONS
Bruce Lipton, The Biology of Belief: Unleashing the Power of Consciousness, Matter and Miracles (Santa Rosa, CA: Elite Books, 2005).

Jurriaan Kamp, "The Honeymoon Effect," Ode Magazine, May/June 2012, <http://odewire.com/honeymooneffect>.

Bruce H Lipton, PhD, "We are not Victims of Heredity," reprinted from James D Baird and Laurie Nadel, Happiness Genes (Franklin Lakes, NJ: New Page Books, 2010), <http://www.creationsmagazine.com/articles/C132/Lipton.html>.

MILDLY ALKALIZING FOODS AND DRINKS
Vinson J, Su X, Zubik L, Bose P, "Phenol Antioxidant Quantity and Quality in Foods: Fruits. J Agric Food Chem 49 (Nov 2001), no 11: 5315–32.

"Exotic Superfoods' Coconut Story," Exotic Superfoods, 2011, <http://www.exoticsuperfoods.com/exotic-superfoods-coconut-story/>.

"Ooh, Scary! The USDA Wants to Protect Us from Raw Almonds," Alliance for Natural Health, Aug 28, 2012, <http://www.anh-usa.org/usda-protect-us-from-raw-almonds/>.

STRONGLY ALKALIZING FOODS AND DRINKS
Ann Wigmore, The Sprouting Book (Wayne, NJ: Avery, 1986), pp 12–13.

ALKALIZING THOUGHTS AND EMOTIONS
M Ted Morter, Jr, Dynamic Health (Rogers, AR: Mortar Health Systems, 1997), p 269.

Mona Lisa Schultz, MD, PhD, "Scientific Results for Affirmations," <http://thebathtubdiva. com/scientific-results-for-affirmations>.

YOU ARE THE CHANGE!

Robert Morse, ND, "Diabetes and Blood Sugar Issues: Part 1," YouTube video, 12:26, posted by DrRobertMorseND, Dec 20, 2011, <http://youtu.be/6T1vBQwJZMo>.

Chapter 9: Nature's Four Fuel Groups

ECODIET FUEL GROUP #1: EARTH
FUEL YOUR BODY THROUGH THE POWER OF PLANT FOODS
Drink Whole Plant-Food Smoothies

Darrell Miller, "Color Wheel of Fruits and Vegetables," Jan 12, 2008, <http://www.disabled-world.com/artman/publish/fruits-vegetables.shtml>.

DRINK SUPERFOOD SMOOTHIES

Kamran Ghasemi, Yosef Ghasemi, and Mohammad Ali Ebra Himza Deh, "Antioxidant Activity, Phenol and Flavonoid Contents of 13 Citrus Species Peels and Tissues," Pak J Pharm Sci 22, no 3 (July 2009): 277–81, <http://www.pjps.pk/CD-PJPS-22-3-09/Paper-7.pdf>.

"The Adventist Health Study: Mortality Studies of Seventh-day Adventists," School of Public Health, Loma Linda University, <http://www.llu.edu/public-health/health/mortality.page>.

"Mung Bean," Sprout People, <http://sproutpeople.org/mung.html>.

You can find more information about Manuka honey at the website of the Active Manuka Honey Association: <http://www.umf.org.nz/>.

Norman W Walker, The Natural Way to Vibrant Health (Prescott, AZ: Norwalk, 1972), p 30.

RAW, LIVING JUICES

Norman W Walker, Fresh Vegetable and Fruit Juices (Prescott: Norwalk, 1970).

You can search for farmers' markets, CSAs, and pick-your-own farms in your area, and buy many products online from family farmers at <www.localharvest.org/csa>.

ECODIET PRINCIPLE #4: PROPER FOOD COMBINING

Herbert M Shelton, Food Combining Made Easy (San Antonio: Willow Pub, 1982). Natural Hygiene was a medical movement that flowered in the 1800s. Herbert Shelton (1895–1984) almost single-handedly revived Natural Hygiene and wrote many books on diet and natural healing. For the many resources of the Natural Hygiene Society, see <http://naturalhygienesociety.org/>.

The Principles Of Digestive Physiology Which Decree Correct Food Combining (various articles), The Science of Raw Food, <http://www.rawfoodexplained.com/digestive-physiology-and-food-combining/index.html>.

ECODIET PRINCIPLE #6: FEASTING AND FASTING

Ori Hofmekler, "New Studies Support the Warrior Diet's Brain Powering and Anti-Aging Effects," Chet Day's Health and Beyond Online, <http://chetday.com/warriordietantiaging.htm>.

Sarah Yang, "Fasting Every Other Day, While Cutting Few Calories, May Reduce Cancer Risk," UC Berkely News, March 14, 2005, <http://www.berkeley.edu/news/media/releases/2005/03/14_intermittentfeeding.shtml>.

BUT WHAT IF I'M HUNGRY?
EAT LIGHT!

Laura Topham, "Why You Get Fatter in Winter … Even Though You Eat LESS," Mail Online, Oct 24, 2011, <http://www.dailymail.co.uk/health/article-2052975/Why-fatter-winter--eat-LESS.html#axzz2Jks3tW8Y>.

ECODIET4KIDS™

"Obesity and Extreme Obesity Rates Decline Among Low-Income Preschool Children," Overweight and Obesity Data and Statistics (Data from the Journal of the AMA), CDC, June 7, 2012, <http://www.cdc.gov/obesity/data/childhood.html>.

Mayo Clinic Staff, "Childhood Obesity," May 4, 2012, <http://www.mayoclinic.com/health/childhood-obesity/DS00698>.

ECODIET FUEL GROUP #2: AIR
FUEL YOUR BODY THROUGH THE POWER OF YOUR BREATH
For more information on conscious breathing, see Dr. Weil's DVD series, Breathing: The Master Key to Self-Healing, <www.drweil.com>. Andrew Weil, MD, is the author of Natural Health, Natural Medicine, and a world-renowned leader and pioneer in the field of integrative medicine.

Sheldon Saul Hendler, MD, PhD, The Oxygen Breakthrough (New York: Morrow, 1989). Dr. Hendler not only brings us the science behind the power of our breath, he outlines breathing exercises that can transform what some call disease when, in fact, what most suffer from is a lack of oxygen.

"The Foundation of Functional Medicine," Optimal Breathing, <http://www.breathing.com/>.

WANT TO LIVE LONGER?
BREATHE!
Paramhansa Yogananda, Autobiography of a Yogi (1946; repr Los Angeles: Self-Realization Fellowship, 1971), p 235.

TRANSFORMATIONAL BREATHING EXERCISES
Dave Scrivens, "Rebounding: Good for the Lymph System," Well Being Journal 17, no 3 (May/June).

Sondra Ray with Markus Ray, "What Is Liberation Breathing®," <https://www.liberationbreathing.com/what-liberation-breathing>. Sondra Ray is a pioneer of Rebirthing breathwork.

ECODIET FUEL GROUP #3: FIRE
FUEL YOUR BODY THROUGH THE POWER OF THE SUN

Irrira Rikki, "Sunlight and the Human Body," August 3, 2008, <http://www.helium.com/items/1135674-photosynthasis-and-the-human-body-the-light-we-live-by>.

EAT LIGHT

Kim Edwards, "Study Shines More Light on Benefit of Vitamin D in Fighting Cancer," UCSD News Center, August 21, 2007, <http://ucsdnews.ucsd.edu/newsrel/health/08-07VitaminDKE-.asp>.

MF Holick, PhD, MD, and Mark Jenkins, The UV Advantage (New York: lbooks, 2003). Dr. Holick is the world's foremost authority on vitamin D and the healing power of natural sunlight. For more information about his research, visit his website at <www.uvadvantage.org>.

Mark Sircus, Ac, OMD, DM(P), "Calcification and Its Treatment with Magnesium and Sodium Thiosulfate," Dec 8, 2009, <http://drsircus.com/medicine/magnesium/calcification-and-its-treatment-with-magnesium-and-sodium-thiosulfate>.

WANT TO BE HEALTHIER?
SUNBATHE!

Jerry Lee Hoover, ND, Natural Medicine, <http://www.free-ebooks.net/ebook/NATURAL->.

MEDICINE

Mark Sircus, "The Secrets of Light," Natural Allopathic Medicine, <http://naturalallopathic.com/cms/index.php?option=com_content&view=article&id=108&Itemid=145>.

WANT TO PROTECT YOUR SKIN?

DRINK YOUR SUNSCREEN

"Sunscreen Dangers," 2004, <http://www.worldimagenaturals.com/blog/archives/000026_ sunscreen_dangers.html>.

FOODS THAT PROTECT YOU

Jorg Mardian, RHN, CPT, MT, CKS, "Foods for Natural Sunscreen Protection," June 17, 2007, <https://healthinmotion.wordpress.com/2007/06/17/foods-for-natural-sunscreen-protection/>.

WANT TO BECOME ENLIGHTENED?

SUNGAZE

TJ White, MA Mainster, PW Wilson, and JH Tips, "Chorioretinal Temperature Increases from Solar Observation," Bulletin of Mathematical Biophysics 33 (1971): 1-17.

Daniel Reid, The Tao of Health, Sex and Longevity (New York: Simon & Schuster, 1989), p 247.

Eat the Sun with Mason Howe Dwinell, directed by Peter Sorcher (Sorcher Films, 2011), DVD.

India's famous sun gazer, Hira Ratan Manek, has lived for extended periods of time solely on light and occasional beverages. His ability to "eat the sun" has been studied by NASA scientists. See his website at <www.solarhealing.com>.

WANT A SLIM, TRIM BODY?

EAT LIGHT

Takako Hara, "Hunger and Eating," Spring 1997, <http://www.csun.edu/~vcpsy00h/students/hunger.htm>.

WANT TO OXYGENATE YOUR BLOOD?

BE A LIGHT ABSORBER

Herbert M Shelton, The Hygienic System 3: Fasting and Sun Bathing (San Antonio: Shelton Health School, 1950).

ECODIET FUEL GROUP #4: WATER
FUEL YOUR BODY THROUGH THE POWER OF WATER

"A Special Interview with Gerald Pollack about Structured Water by Dr. Mercola," January 2011, transcript available at <http://mercola.fileburst.com/PDF/Expert InterviewTranscripts/Interview-Pollack-Interview-structured-water.pdf>.

F Batmanghelidg, MD, Your Body's Many Cries for Water, 2nd Ed (Falls Church, VA: Global Solutions Inc, 1997).

THE NEW SCIENCE OF STRUCTURED WATER

Hippocrates (400 BCE), On Airs, Waters, and Places, trans by Francis Adams, <http://classics.mit.edu/Hippocrates/airwatpl.1.1.html>.

Dr. Mu Shik Jhon, The Water Puzzle and the Hexagonal Key, trans (from Korean) and ed by MJ Pangman (Uplifting Press, Inc, 2004), p 29.

Clayton Nolte, personal communications, July 2012.

Dr. Gerald Polluck, Professor of Bioengineering, "Water, Energy, and Life: Fresh Views from the Water's Edge," 32nd Annual Faculty Lecture, University of Washington, video uploaded by UWTV on April 29, 2009, <http://www.youtube.com/watch?v=XVBEwn6iWOo>.

"A Special Interview with Gerald Pollack by Dr. Mercola," <http://mercola.fileburst.com/PDF/ExpertInterviewTranscripts/Interview-Pollack-Interview-structured-water.pdf>.

WANT TO PREVENT INFLAMMATION IN YOUR BODY?
FILTER YOUR TAP WATER

"Over 300 Pollutants in US Tap Water," Environmental Working Group, Dec 2009, <http://www.ewg.org/tap-water/home>.

Samantha Chang, "Dr. Deepak Chopra Discusses the Role Toxins Play in Breast Cancer and Obesity," Sept 2012, <http://www.examiner.com/article/dr-deepak-chopra-discusses-the-role-toxins-play-breast-cancer-and-obesity>.

Joseph Mercola, MD, "Lead Poisoning Alert: This Widely Used Drink Is Dangerous," Nov 12, 2011, <http://articles.mercola.com/sites/articles/archive/2011/11/12/jeff-green-on-fluoride-part-1.aspx>.

John Yiamouyiannis, PhD, in an interview with Gary Null, March 1995, referenced in Gary Null, "The Fluoridation Fiasco," Townsend Letter for Doctors and Patients, <http://www.tldp.com/issue/157-8/157fluor.htm>.

John Yiamouyiannis, Fluoride the Aging Factor: How to Recognize and Avoid the Devastating Effects of Fluoride, 3rd Ed (Delaware, OH: Health Action Pr, 1993).

Lynn Landes, "Alzheimer's in America: The Aluminum-Phosphate Fertilizer Connection," Aug 19, 2002, <http://www.commondreams.org/views02/0819-06.htm>.

Robert Carton, PhD, former scientist with the US EPA, interviewed on CBC TV's "Marketplace" on November 24, 1992, referenced in Gene Shaparenko, "Pure Drinking Water and the Immune System," <http://www.aquatechnology.net/immune_system.html>.

J. William Hirzy, PhD, "Why EPA Headquarters Union of Scientists Opposes Fluoridation," prepared on behalf of the National Treasury Employees Union Chapter 280, US EPA, <http://www.nteu280.org/Issues/Fluoride/NTEU280-Fluoride.htm>.

WANT TO BE HEALTHIER?
DON'T TREAT THIRST WITH MEDICATION!

Batmanghelidg, Your Body's Many Cries for Water, p 67.

Polluck, "Water, Energy, and Life: Fresh Views from the Water's Edge," <http://www.youtube.com/watch?v=XVBEwn6iWOo>.

WANT A SLIM, TRIM BODY?
YOU'RE NOT HUNGRY, YOU'RE THIRSTY!

Leroy R Perry, Jr, "Think You're Drinking Enough Water?" condensed from PARADE Magazine, <http://www.naturodoc.com/library/nutrition/water.htm>.

F. Batmanghelidg, Your Body's Many Cries for Water, pp 99–100.

Wayne Scott Anderson, MD, Dr A's Habits of Health, (Annapolis, MD: Habits of Health Press,2008), pp 114–15; pub March 6, 2012, in "Water, Nature's Gift," <http://www.drwayneandersen.com/2012/03/06/water-natures-gift-2/>.

WANT TO PREVENT AGING?
DRINK STRUCTURED WATER

"A Special Interview with Gerald Pollack," <http://mercola.fileburst.com/PDF/ExpertInterviewTranscripts/Interview-Pollack-Interview-structured-water.pdf>.

SEARCHING FOR PEAK PERFORMANCE?
CHARGE YOUR WATER BATTERIES

Martin Fox, "Water: the Essential Nutrient," in Healthy Water, Internet Health Library, <http://www.internethealthlibrary.com/Environmental-Health/WaterTheEssential Nutrient.htm>.

"A Special Interview with Gerald Pollack," <http://mercola.fileburst.com/PDF/ExpertInterviewTranscripts/Interview-Pollack-Interview-structured-water.pdf>.

THE POWER OF COLONIC HYDROTHERAPY

"Death Begins in the Colon," Natural Healing Forum, <http://curezone.com/forums/am.asp?i=1846920>.

Diana Schwarzbein, MD, "GI Overview," <http://www.schwarzbeinprinciple.com/pgs/testing/testing_overvw_gi.html>.

Bernard Jensen, DC, ND, PhD, Dr. Jensen's Guide to Better Bowel Care: A Complete Program for Tissue Cleansing through Bowel Management (New York: Avery, 1999), p 11.

See Richard Anderson's Cleanse and Purify Thyself book series from Christobe.

USE YOUR MIND AND EMOTIONS TO STRUCTURE YOUR INTERNAL WATERS

Masaru Emoto, The Hidden Messages in Water (Hillsboro, OR: Beyond Words Pub, 2004).

Dr. Leonard Coldwell, "The Secret Info," <http://www.worldhealthnation.com>.

"Dr. Leonard Coldwell, "Every Cancer Can be Cured in Weeks explains Dr. Leonard Coldwell," video uploaded by iHealthTube on Nov 28, 2011, <http://www.youtube.com/watch?v=DgbdNNfotwM>.

CHAPTER 10: CONCLUSION

THE INVISIBLE INFLUENCE OF YOUR DIET ON THE EARTH

Ryan, John, and Durning, Alan, Stuff: The Secret Lives of Everyday Things (Seattle: Northwest Environment Watch, 1997), p 55.

John Robbins, The Food Revolution: How Your Diet Can Help Save Your Life and Our World (San Francisco, CA: Red Wheel/Weiser LLC, 2011), Kindle edition, p 267.

David Wilcock, "2012 Event Horizon: Prophecies and Science of a Golden Age," video uploaded by DavidWilcock333 on May 3, 2010, <http://www.youtube.com/watch?v=cEyqT2_ricA>.

John Robbins, The Food Revolution, Kindle edition, p 236.

J Fillip, "American Farmers and USDA Start to Take Organic Seriously," Not Man Apart (Friends of the Earth Newsmagazine), September 1980.

For the Meatless Monday movement, see <http://www.meatlessmonday.com/why-meatless/>.

Robbins, The Food Revolution, p 290.

Lucy Sandbach, "Nitrogen—The Bad Guy of Global Warming," March 21, 2007, The Naked Scientists, Cambridge University, <http://www.thenakedscientists.com/HTML/features/article/nitrogenthebadguyofglobalwarming1160583306/>.

RESOURCES

Organic-Biodynamic Produce

Community Support Agriculture (CSA)
7200 Wisconsin Avenue
Suite 601
Bethesda, Maryland 20814
1-800-843-7751
www.csa.com

Diamond Organics
The Organic Food Catalog
P.O. Box 2159
Freedom, California 95019
1-888-674-2642
www.diamondorganics.com

Green Polka Box
www.tonitoney.com

Ocean Grown, Inc.
7453 Commercial Circle
Ft. Pierce, Florida 34951
1-941-921-2401
www.oceangrown.com

The Tower Garden
www.tonitoney.com

Whitted Bowers Fruit Farm
8707 Art Road
Cedar Grove, North Carolina 27231
1-919-732-5132
www.whittedbowersfarm@mac.com

Organic Raw Foods

Active Manuka Honey and Royal Jelly
CalComp Nutrition Inc.
2021 Clay Pike, Suite 1
Irwin, PA 15642
1-877-919-9992

Brad's Raw Chips
P. O. Box 210
Pipersville, PA 18947
1-215-766-3739
www.bradsrawchips.com

Celtic Sea Salt®
Selina Naturally
4 Celtic Drive, Arden NC 28704
1-800-867-7258

Great American Wholefood Farmacy
117 E. Main Street
Rogersville, Tennessee 37857
1-423-921-7848
www.wholefoodfarmacy.com

Jaffe Brothers
28560 Lilac Road
Valley Center, California 92082
1-760-749-1133

Living Qi Organic Matcha Green Tea
Living Qi LLC
1-877-544-2583
www.living-qi.com
Matt Monarch
www.therawfoodworld.com

Sunfood Nutrition
11655 Riverside Drive
Lakeside, California 92040
1-800-205-2350
www.sunfood.com

Sun Organic Farm
P.O. Box 409
San Marcos, California 92079
1-888-269-9888
www.sunorganic.com

UliMana, Inc.
P.O. Box 18058
Asheville, North Carolina 28814
1-828-713-3469
www.ulimana.com

Wilderness Family Naturals
1-800-945-3801
www.wildernessfamilynaturals.com

Supplements

Hallelujah Acres
900 S. Post Road
Shelby, North Carolina 28152
1-704-481-1700
www.hacres.com

Health Force Nutritionals
1835A S. Centre City Pkwy. #411
Escondido, California 92025
1-800-357-2717
www.healthforce.com

Morter Health Systems
215 West Poplar
Rogers, Arkansas 72756
1-800-874-1478
www.morterhealthsystem.com

Seven Point2
The Alkaline Company
www.tonitoney.com

The Synergy Company
2279 South Resource Boulevard
Moab, Utah 84532
1-800-723-0277
www.thesynergycompany.com

Synergistic Nutrition
Stephen Heuer
1-864-895-6250
www.sgn80.com

Intestinal Cleansing and Probiotics

Arise and Shine
Richard Anderson, ND
562 Parsons Drive
Medford, Oregon 97501
1-800-688-2444
www.ariseandshine.com

Candida, Parasites, Heavy Metal Detox
www.tonitoney.com

EcoDiet Kitchen Equipment

BlendTec
www.tonitoney.com

Excalibur Dehydrators
www.tonitoney.com

Hurom Juicer
www.tonitoney.com

Water Systems
www.tonitoney.com

Holistic Healing Clinics

Alternative Cancer Clinic
Saint Joseph Medical Center
Dr. Rogers and Dr. Rayes
www.doctorofhope.com

Brain Longevity Center
Lorne Label, MD
2100 Lynn Road, Suite 230
Thousand Oaks, California 91360
1-805-497-4500
www.cns-neurology.com

The Cleanse Club
Asheville, NC
www.tonitoney.com

Hippocrates Health Institute
1443 Palmdale Court
West Palm Beach, Florida 33411
1-800-842-2125
www.hippocratesinst.org

O3 Institute & EcoSpa
Dr. Teo Tomas, Founder
Delicas, Costa Rica
(506) 2640-0824 or (506) 2640- 0893
www.o3institute.com

Optimum Health Institute
6970 Central Avenue
Lemon Grove, California 91945
1-800-993-4325
www.optimumhealth.org

Paracelsus Biological Clinic
Thomas Rau, MD
c/o The Marion Institute
3 Barnabas Road
Marion, Massachusetts 02738
1-508-748-0816

Path to Health
Dave Carpenter, ND
Idaho Falls, Idaho
1-208-529-0384
www.pathtohealth.com

Tennant Institute for Integrative Medicine
Jerry Tennant, MD
9901 East Valley Ranch Parkway, #1015
Irving, Texas 75063
1-866-612-4461
www.tennantinstitute.com

Tree of Life Rejuvenation Center
Gabriel Cousens, MD
P.O. Box 778
Patagonia, Arizona 85624
1-866-394-2520
www.treeoflife.nu

The Wellness Clinic
Robert Jones, Director
Green Creek, NC
1-828-863-4794

Holistic Denistry

Robert Chan, DDS
Suite 11, 2425 East Street
Concord, CA 94520-1926
1-925-363-3902

Stephen R. Evans, DDS
16427 FM 344W
Bullard, TX 75757
1-903-825-7400

Gary McCown, DDS
2923 Alcoa Highway
Knoxville, TN37920
Phone: (865) 579-3762

Darick Nordstrom, DDS
930 Sunnyslope Road, Suite D4
Hollister, CA 95023
1-831-637-1675

Custom Nutrition and Blood Testing

American Metabolic Testing Laboratory
Emile Schandle, Ph.D.
1818 Sheridan Street #102
Hollywood, Florida 33020
1-954-929-4814

Forgiveness and Emotional Healing

Energetic Clearing Process
Judith Johnson
329 Eden Drive
Hillsborough, North Carolina
1-919-241-3151
www.energeticclearingprocess.com

Heartland Teaching Center
Dr. Michael Ryce
Theodosia, Missouri 65761
1-417-273-4838
www.Iforgive.net

Institute of HeartMath®
14700 West Park Ave.,
Boulder Creek, California 95006
1-800-711-6221

Rebirthing Breathwork
Sondra Ray, Rebirther
www.sondraray.com

Recommended Reading

*Anti-Arthritis, Anti-Inflammation
Cookbook: Healing Though Natural Foods*
Author: Gary Null, Ph.D.
www.essentialpublishing,org/bookstore

Breathing: The Master Key to Self Healing
Author: Andrew Weil, MD
www.drweil.com

Cancer is a Fungus
Author: Dr. Tullio Simoncini
www.cancerisafungus.com

Cleanse and Purify Thyself
Author: Dr. Richard Anderson
P.O. Box 1643
Medford, Oregon 97501
1-800-688-2444

Conscious Language
Author: Robert Tennyson Stevens
352 Depot Street, Suite 210
Asheville, North Carolina 28801
1-828-258-2220
www.masterysystems.com

*Dr. Neal Barnard's Program for Reversing
Diabetes*
Author: Neal Barnard, MD
www.nealbarnard.org

Farmacist Desk Reference
Author: Don Tolman
www.dontolman.com

Green for Life
Author: Victoria Boutenko
The Raw Family
Ashland, Oregon 975520
www.rawfamily.com

Healing is Voltage
Author: Jerry Tennant, MD
9901 East Valley Ranch Parkway, #1015
Irving, Texas 75063
1-866-612-4461
www.tennantinstitute.com

My Big Toe
Thomas Campbell
www.mybigtoe.com

Rainbow Green Live-Food Cuisine
Author: Gabriel Cousens, MD
Tree of Life Rejuvenation Center
P.O. Box 778
Patagonia, Arizona 85624
1-866-394-2520
www.treeoflife.nu

Reverse Arthritis and Pain Naturally: A Proven Approach to a Pain-Free Life
Author: Gary Null, Ph.D.
www.essentialpublishing,org/bookstore

Spontaneous Evolution
Authors: Bruce Lipton, Ph.D.
Steve Bhaerman
www.wakeuplaughing.com

Superfoods: The Food and Medicine of the Future
Author: David Wolfe
www.davidwolfe.com

The 80-10-10 Diet
Author: Dr. Doug Graham
www.douggraham.com

The Biology of Belief
Author: Bruce Lipton, Ph.D.
www.brucelipton.com

The China Study
Author T. Colin Campbell
www.thechinastudy.com

The Complete Encyclopedia of Natural Healing
Author: Gary Null, Ph.D.
www.garynull.com

The Curse of Louis Pasteur
Author: Nancy Appleton, Ph.D.
P.O. Box 3083
Santa Monica, California 90403
www.nancyappleton.com

The Food Revolution
Author: John Robbins
www.foodrevolution.org

The Germ that Causes Cancer
Author: Doug Kaufmann
www.knowthecause.com

The Swiss Secret to Optimal Health
Author: Dr. Thomas Rau, MD
Paracelsus Biological Medicine Network
3 Barnabas Road
Marion, Massachusetts 02738
1-508-748-0816

The UV Advantage
Michael F. Holick, MD
715 Albany Street, M-1013
Boston, MA 02118
1-617-638-4545

Why is this Happening to me AGAIN?
Dr. Michael Ryce
Route 3; Box 3280
Theodosia, Missouri 65761
1-417-273-4838
www.whyagain.com

Your Health Your Choice
Author: Dr. Ted Morter, Jr.
215 West Poplar
Rogers, Arkansas 72756
1-800-874.-478
www.morter.com

ESSENTIAL
PUBLISHING

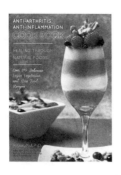

Anti-Arthritis, Anti-Inflammation Cookbook: Healing Through Natural Foods
by Gary Null, Ph.D.

This *New York Times* best-selling author brings you more than 270 anti-arthritis, anti-inflammation recipes to heal conditions and diseases of inflammation, which are largely perpetuated by the high-fat, high-sugar, chemically laden Standard American Diet (S.A.D.). Prevent and reverse diseases like arthritis, cancer, diabetes and heart disease by making the delicious offerings within this book the mainstay of a new eating program...your health and life depend on it!

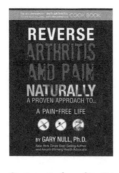

Reverse Arthritis & Pain Naturally: A proven approach to an anti-inflammatory, pain-free life
by Gary Null, Ph.D.

Arthritis is the most common cause of disability in the United States today, limiting the activities of a remarkable 50 million adults. Like cancer, diabetes and heart disease, arthritis is a disease of inflammation rooted in lifestyle choices. This book takes an in-depth look at the epidemic of arthritis and chronic pain sweeping our nation today, providing an explanation for its causes while offering a proven lifestyle protocol to reverse and prevent them naturally.

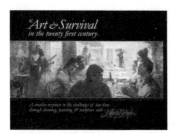

Art & Survival in the 21st Century: A creative response to the challenges of our time through drawing, painting & sculpture
by James Menzel Joseph

This art and social criticism book takes a profound look at the role of art in humanity's survival, and features over 200 exquisite and beautiful paintings and drawings of James Menzel Joseph, celebrated award-winning artist, author master art teacher, and activist.

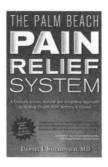

The Palm Beach Pain Relief System: A Clinically-proven, Natural and Integrative Approach to Healing Chronic Pain, Arthritis & Injury
by Daniel Nuchovich, M.D.

This comprehensive, revolutionary, proven medical treatment program utilizes natural therapies, including the whole-foods Mediterranean Diet, to overcome chronic pain. This drug-free, integrative approach is working for 90+% of patients suffering from arthritis, and other diseases of information. Avoid unnecessary surgeries and free yourself from the potentially deadly trap of unsuccessful pharmaceutical-based therapies.

ESSENTIAL PUBLISHING

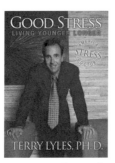

Good Stress: Living Younger Longer
by Terry Lyles, Ph.D.

Seeing stress as good is essential for achieving a youthful and vibrant life, says Dr. Terry Lyles, in this groundbreaking book inspired by years of rescue work at some the world's worst disasters: 9/11, Hurricane Katrina and the tsunami in Thailand. Dr. Lyles, known as America's Stress Doctor, implores us to see stress as a benevolent force. "If you want to live younger longer, start now by seeing stress for what it really is – a catalyst for positive growth and change.

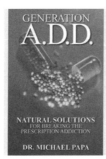

Generation A.D.D.: Natural Solutions for Breaking the Prescription Addiction
by Dr. Michael Papa

Free yourself and your children from the bonds of chemical dependency! In this timely and important book, Dr. Michael Papa urges us to explore and understand the symptoms and underlying causes of ADD/ADHD, and to choose natural solutions first, offering numerous approaches that have worked successfully with patients over the years.

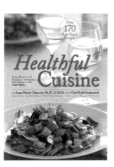

Healthful Cuisine – 2nd Edition
by Anna Maria Clement, Ph.D., N.M.D, L.N.C. and Kelly Serbonich

Learn about the superior health and nutritional benefits of raw and living foods from the world's #1 medical spa, Hippocrates Health Institute. This book contains: 150 raw and living food recipes, 40 pages of illustrated raw food preparation techniques, and more than 50 full-color photographs showing step-by-step instructions, plus tips from the experts. Making healthy raw foods has never been so easy.

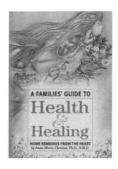

A Families Guide to Health & Healing: Home Remedies from the Heart
by Anna Maria Clement, Ph.D., N.M.D, L.N.C.

Bring healing back into the home! In this beautifully illustrated full color book, Dr. Anna Maria Clement, co-director of the world-famous Hippocrates Health Institute, show us how easy it can be to heal naturally with herbs, natural therapies, baths, flower remedies and aromatherapy. Contains more than 40 years of time-tested, clinical experience with natural healing modalities.

INDEX

8

A

B

C

oxygen *(continued)*
 cells and, 27, 36, 160
 chemicals and, 124
 chlorophyll and, 136
 disease and, 35
 environment and, 146
 fats and, 109
 health and, 207, 209
 human body and, 12
 internal environment and, 13-14, 17, 25,
  28, 35, 37, 39, 49, 79, 104, 117, 146
 internal exchange, 208
 internal water and, 13
 lack of, results from, 26
 necessity of, 208
 oils and, 107
 our bodies and, 208
 oxidation and, 42
 pH and, 13, 43
 rancidity and, 108
 respiration and, 35
 water and, 208, 223, 229, 232

P

Paracelsus Clinic, 11
paradigm scale, 243
Pasteur, Louis, 3, 238
pasteurization, 74-75, 82, 135
pasteurized food(s), 74-75, 88, 114, 135, 153,
 184
Pelasgians, The, 62
Pepsi, 85, 96, 123-124
Perfect Health Diet, 68
pesticides, 42, 75-77, 80, 96, 100, 125
 foods and, 80-81
pH, 13, 29, 39-45, 49-54, 66, 106, 108, 113, 122-
 125, 131, 135, 138, 140, 232, 238-239, 243, 246
 saliva test and, 53
 urine tests and, 51
pharmaceuticals. *See* drug(s)
Philochorus, 62
phosphates, 26-27, 64, 66, 94-95
phthalates, 125
phytochemical(s), 130
phytonutrient(s), 15, 65, 93, 99, 133, 147-150,
 154, 170, 207
phytotoxins, 64, 129
Pineapple Coconut Watercress Smoothie, 185

Pineapple Gazpacho Soup, 189
Pitchford, Paul, 130
Plum Good Cream Sauce, 202
Plutarch, 61
Pollack, Gerald, PhD, 222, 224, 227, 229-230
Pollan, Michael, 94
polyunsaturated oils, 107-108, 111
Potato Corn Soup, 200
Potato Leek Soup, 201
processed food(s), 2-3, 27-28, 37, 43, 53, 93-94,
 97, 104-105, 107, 112-113, 147, 163-164, 168,
 173, 203
processed meat(s), 27, 68, 71
producer organisms, 14-15
protein, 66-67, 75, 90, 93, 96-98, 118, 129, 150,
 157-158, 205-206, 227
Pusztai, Arpad, 83

Q

QAI, 80

R

radiation, 72
Radicchio Pear Salad, 197
rainforest, 41
 inner. *See* inner rainforest
RAW SALADS, 188
 Apple Juice Dressing, 191
 Great Greek Salad, 190
 Italian Kale Salad, 190
 Oil-Free Pesto, 192
 Sweet and Sour Dressing, 192
 Watercress Papaya Salad, 191
 Winter Root Salad, 191
 Zucchini Linguini Pesto Salad, 192
RAW SOUPS, 188
 Gazpacho Avocado Soup, 188
 Pineapple Gazpacho Soup, 189
 Thai Coconut Soup, 189
 Tomato Basil Soup, 188
RAW WRAPS, 188
 Fig Fuji Salsa Wrap, 193
 Fruit Salsa Wrap, 193
raw, living foods, 146, 153
Red Raspberry Dressing, 196
reducer organisms, 14, 19, 26, 42, 44, 101
 candida, 30

Welcome
to the Alkaline Movement

Become part of the next major shift in the wellness industry...

THE ALKALINE MOVEMENT.

The First Company in History to

Make it SIMPLE and EASY to Alkalize Your Body

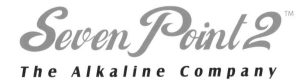

Seven Point 2™

The Alkaline Company

Seven Point 2 ™

The Alkaline Company

It's no secret, chronic health conditions are on the rise because of poor nutrition. It's not just saturated fats, sugars, and preservatives in our food, it's that so much of our foods are acidic!

Numerous studies show a direct link between acidic pH levels in the human body and chronic, and sometimes terminal, illness. Research shows evidence that sickness and disease thrive in an acidic environment. Become more alkaline by opting for a plant based "green" diet leading to a healthier body and mind. We believe it's time to make pH balance a priority for everyone. This is why we created the SevenPoint2 line of products. They are designed to get you alkaline and keep you there. SevenPoint2 is here to prove it can be accomplished without a fad diet or enduring horrible tasting supplements.

We are dedicated to making alkalinity a fundamental concept in the wellness industry by distributing our products to the millions of people interested in attaining optimal health. Finally, becoming alkaline is made simple (and delicious) with SevenPoint2.

The typical American diet is high in acid forming foods, which causes our bodies to become more susceptible to disease. Is it any wonder that chronic health conditions are on the rise at an alarming rate?

The First Company in History to Make it SIMPLE and EASY to Alkalize Your Body

Health: The Fires Within

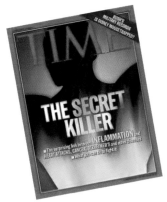

Do you know the effects of chronic inflammation?

Time Magazine published an article entitled, Health: The Fires Within, about the dangerous effects on our health from chronic inflammation. This story was so groundbreaking in the fields of medical and nutritional science that it warranted being the cover story. Here is a chilling excerpt from that article: "Inflammation has become one of the hottest areas of medical research. Hardly a week goes by without the publication of yet another study uncovering a new way that chronic inflammation does harm to the body. In other words, chronic inflammation may be the engine that drives many of the most feared illnesses of middle and old age.

"This concept is so intriguing because it suggests a new and possibly a much simpler way of warding off disease."
- Time Magazine

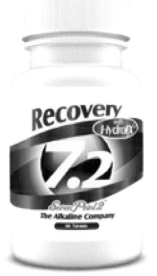

Recovery with HydroFx, the first ever, all natural, molecular hydrogen, super anti-inflammatory.

A Scientific Breakthrough!

7.2 Recovery with HydroFX™

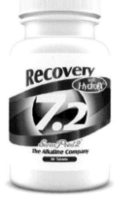

Recovery with HydroFX is comprised of a unique blend of redox-active, hydrogen-generating alkaline minerals. This breakthrough proprietary formula has been clinically tested to release molecular hydrogen, produce a negative oxidation reduction potential, create an anti-acid, alkalizing effect and to increase cellular hydration. The most notable benefit is its ability to release such a significant amount of molecular hydrogen (H2).

Alkalizing: Effectively neutralizes excess acids in bodies of all types including lactic acid.

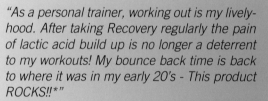

"As a personal trainer, working out is my livelyhood. After taking Recovery regularly the pain of lactic acid build up is no longer a deterrent to my workouts! My bounce back time is back to where it was in my early 20's - This product ROCKS!!*"

— Mike Z.

Helps to

- Reduce Inflammation
- Reduce Joint Discomfort
- Reduce Lactic Acid
- Increase Energy
- Anti-Aging
- Cardio-Protective
- Neuro-Protective
- Intestinal Protection
- Skin Rejuvenation
- Increased Stamina
- And Much More*

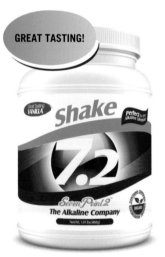

GREAT TASTING!

21g of Plant Based Protein

7.2 Shake

This great tasting vegan shake is the foundation of your alkaline lifestyle. The SevenPoint2™ Shake's proprietary formula is an excellent high quality, low carbohydrate protein source. This easily digestible formula is high in fiber and provides an extensive array of naturally occurring amino acids which are the building blocks of protein. This low glycemic, high performance vegetarian superfood, assists your body in burning fat and becoming alkaline all at the same time!

√ Organic
√ Vegan
√ Kosher
√ Sugar-Free
√ Non-GMO
√ Gluten Free
√ Soy Free
√ Dairy Free
√ Nut Free

This is by far the best tasting shake I have ever had. It is so clean with regards to the ingredients. I took it in for my family doctor to see and he was impressed. *

— Laura H., Ca.

7.2 Greens

SevenPoint2™ Organic Greens are a delicious and revitalizing essential supplement designed to gently detoxify the body and help you achieve an alkaline lifestyle.

Our greens are loaded with healthy green superfoods, cereal grasses and alkalizing vegetables in a great tasting powder. Unlike other green products commonly associated with an unfavorable taste, our greens taste so good that even the most finicky palates will enjoy them. They really do taste that good!

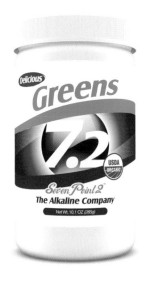

"These are the best tasting greens. My entire family loves them and that makes me feel better, especially since it's hard to get our children to eat lots of greens. SevenPoint2 Greens provide the best nutrition for us all!" *

- BROOKE B., Ca.

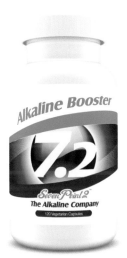

7.2 Alkaline Booster

We have affectionately nicknamed our Alkaline Booster, "The Hall Pass!" After having an acidic meal and/or beverage(s) or before bed, this product works instantly to bring you from acidic pH levels to alkaline. The SevenPoint2™ Alkaline Booster allows you to live the lifestyle you are accustomed to while staying on track with your goal of being pH balanced.

"I've had major digestive issues for years that have really affected my life. I noticed a huge improvement in just a couple of days using these Alkaline Boosters! I love them and take them every day!"

- JASON M., Ca.

Seven Point 2 ™
The Alkaline Company

Visit our website for information about our Fast Track Programs to Alkalinity:
- 30 Days to Alkalinity - Made Simple and Easy
- Seven Week Alkaline Weight Loss Transformation

7.2 Green Caps

The SevenPoint2™ Green Caps
are a revitalizing essential supplement,
designed to feed your body the nutrients it needs
and to help you achieve an alkaline lifestyle.
Our Green Caps are loaded with plenty of
healthy green superfoods,
cereal grasses and alkalizing vegetables.

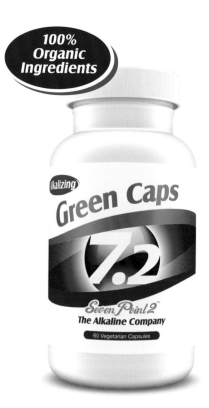

100% Organic Ingredients

Feel Great Now!

✓ *Contains only organic ingredients*
✓ *100% Whole food, non-GMO, vegan nutrition*
✓ *Highly alkalizing*
✓ *Convenient, easy to swallow capsule*
✓ *Naturally energizing*
✓ *Certified Kosher*
✓ *Gluten free, dairy free, soy free, nut free, nightshade free, sugar free, and free of all artificial ingredients*

Seven Point 2™
The Alkaline Company

*These statements have not been evaluated by the Food and Drug Administration. This product is not intended to diagnose, treat, cure or prevent any disease.

The Seven Week Alkaline Weight Loss Transformation

Fat Loss + Lean Muscle = Transformation

Welcome to the SevenPoint2 Alkaline Weight Loss Transformation. NOT another fad diet. NOT another brutal workout program. Real change based on real science and basic human physiology. Trans-for-ma-tion (noun) def., "a seemingly miraculous change in appearance."

Most people, at some time in their lives, have tried a diet. The biggest challenge is that while most traditional weight-loss plans can help you lose weight, they can many times make your health worse by causing your body to become too acidic. This, in turn, can cause a major disruption in your metabolism, so even if you do lose weight, you end up gaining it back even faster.

How the Transformation works is simple, and the key is alkalinity. When you eat acidic foods, it sends the body into a "fight or flight" response causing it to store the excess acid as fat. When you eat alkaline foods, your body tends to emulsify fat (takes big fat and turns it into little fat) making it easier for the body to further digest and eliminate. This one fundamental key, coupled with the breakthrough concept of "Nutrient Timing," is what makes the SevenPoint2 Alkaline Weight Loss Transformation the ONLY program of its type to produce REAL, lasting change.

Experience for yourself what Hollywood A-List celebrities and professional athletes have discovered. Visit us at www.SevenPoint2.com and learn what the SevenPoint2 Alkaline Weight Loss Transformation can do for you.

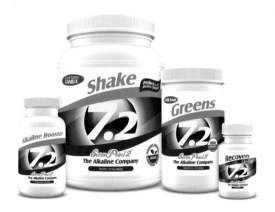

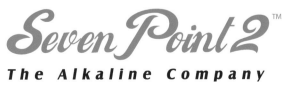

The Alkaline Company

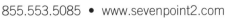

855.553.5085 • www.sevenpoint2.com

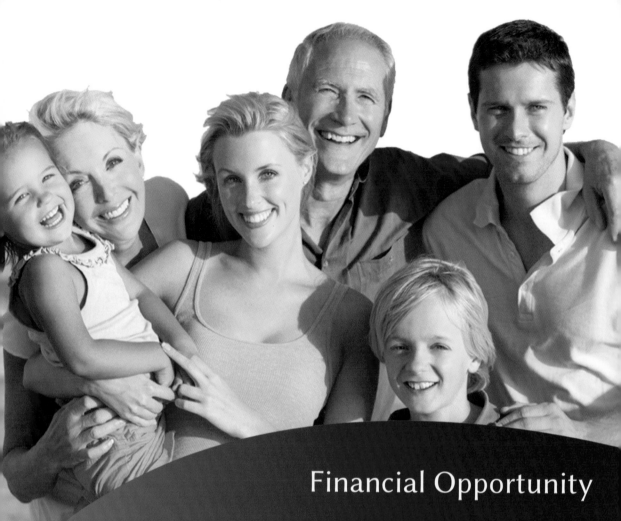

Financial Opportunity

SevenPoint2 was created to be the next billion dollar brand, leading the way in The Alkaline Movement.

This is one of the most important missions of our time, and experts are predicting this to be the wave of the future. Paul Zane Pilzer, world renowned economist and author of "The Wellness Revolution", calls Health and Wellness the next trillion dollar industry. Although still ground floor, The Alkaline Movement is becoming the largest shift in the history of the Wellness Industry.

This truly is the opportunity of a lifetime which has allowed SevenPoint2 to create a powerful financial plan for people who would like to promote our products. Our proven business model is simple and we have a training system that allows everyone the opportunity to succeed. Simply fill out our distributor card to receive more information on how you can lock in your legacy position with SevenPoint2, The Alkaline Company.